C000148419

LIVING THERAPY

Counselling for Problem Gambling

Person-Centred Dialogues

Richard Bryant-Jefferies

Radcliffe Publishing

Oxford • Seattle

Radcliffe Publishing Ltd
18 Marcham Road
Abingdon
Oxon OX14 1AA
United Kingdom

www.radcliffe-oxford.com
Electronic catalogue and worldwide online ordering facility.

British Library Cataloguing in Publication Data

A catalogue record for this book is available from the British Library.

ISBN 1 85775 740 8

Typeset by Aarontype Ltd, Easton, Bristol
Printed and bound by TJ International Ltd, Padstow, Cornwall

Contents

Foreword

In 1987 when I began my PhD on slot machine gambling, little did I know that almost two decades later I would still find myself irresistibly hooked into researching a fascinating and interesting area of human behaviour. The academic study – and to some extent treatment – of gambling has come a long way in 20 years. Given the paucity of data in the area, I managed to create a productive niche for myself and have spent much of my time trying to bring in and facilitate other researchers and practitioners to the area.

Since the introduction of the National Lottery in 1994, gambling in the UK has become more destigmatised and more demasculinised. People's attitudes towards gambling have softened and gambling is now seen as a socially acceptable leisure activity rather than a sin or a vice. The new Gambling Bill that was passed by Parliament in April 2005 will almost certainly lead to more opportunities and access to gambling in the UK than we have ever seen before. If we are not already a nation of gamblers then we soon will be! The downside of deregulation is that more people will gamble. As a consequence, there will be a growing number of gambling 'casualties', some of whom will want professional intervention and treatment.

Over the last decade, I have been relentless in trying to get gambling addiction on the mental health agenda and have argued that gambling in its most excessive forms can be just as destructive as any other form of addictive behaviour for the individual. In the UK, there are so few practitioners who are aware that gambling can be a problem. There are only a handful of people who even specialise in the treatment of gambling problems.

I was therefore delighted to be asked to write a foreword to Richard Bryant-Jefferies' book. Books on the treatment of problem gamblers have been few and far between especially when compared to other more traditional addictions. What's more, of the few that have been written, many are either too dry and academic, or too therapeutically lightweight to be of real use to counsellors, therapists and other practitioners. That is why I am delighted that Richard has written this book.

Richard has an engaging writing style and this book is written in such a way that most readers will be able to follow his very accessible style of writing. Whether you are a treatment practitioner, a researcher, scholar, or someone with a passing interest in the study of gambling, there is something for everyone in this book. Although I am a psychologist, I am not a practitioner – yet Richard's vibrant text is a good advert for taking up the role of therapist and helper. The book aims to bring the therapeutic process alive and this is something that Richard has achieved.

One of the unique aspects of this book is the format. Richard helps bring to life the gamblers in treatment through the innovative use of two very detailed (fictional) case studies. As Richard points out, he doesn't provide all the answers, but he does highlight the mind set of a typical problem gambler. Any of us who have worked with problem gamblers over the years will recognise both 'Max' and 'Rob'. I have never read a book (or journal paper) in this area that is so detailed and reflective as the one you are reading now.

I wish Richard every success with the book and hope that readers will find it as stimulating and 'experiential' a read as I did.

Professor Mark Griffiths
Professor of Gambling Studies
Division of Psychology
Nottingham Trent University
May 2005

Foreword

As a former, and sometimes lapsed, slot-machine addict, I am delighted to be writing a foreword to Richard Bryant-Jefferies' latest addition to the *Living Therapy* series. It may seem strange to say, but during my teens and early twenties, some of the most pleasurable moments in my life involved standing in front of a slot-machine, cigarette in one hand and pint of beer (ideally) in the other, listening to the clatter of coins coming out of the pay-out chute. I remember, one day, thinking that this was what heaven must be like: pleasure, pleasure and more pleasure ... a wonderfully warm glow of relief, excitement and accomplishment all wrapped up into one. Much more common, however, were the feelings of shame, self-hatred and remorse that almost inevitably followed a bout of slot-machine playing when, ten or more pounds worse off, I would slink away from the arcade or pub feeling sick to my teeth.

It is probably not an understatement to say that, at times, I left the machines feeling like I wanted to end it all. It was not just the burning sensations of self-hatred and remorse, it was also the sense that, expelled from the world of flashing lights, 'holds' and 'nudges', nothing seemed to matter. Everything else was grey and limp by comparison. Often, it would take me an hour or more to re-engage with the world and others. I just didn't care.

At those times, it never occurred to me to talk to anyone about my problems. I desperately wanted to overcome my addiction, but felt far too ashamed to discuss it with family or friends. I assumed, probably rightly, that they would tell me how stupid I was and how much money I was wasting, and there was already enough of that criticism going on in my head. Besides which, I didn't really believe that they would be able to help me. It was just for me and my best friend, then, who also moved in and out of gambling addictions, to try and find our own solutions to our problems: most of which failed the moment we walked past an 'amusement' arcade with more than a fiver in our pockets.

Ironically, perhaps, I also did not discuss my slot-machine addiction with the handful of therapists that I saw during that period in my life. Partly, no doubt, out of sheer embarrassment over the sums of money I was squandering; but also, perhaps, out of a sense that these very sensible, slightly reserved adults could never really understand the excitement and 'glamour' that drew me towards the slot-machines. In this sense, Richard Bryant-Jefferies has done the counselling and psychotherapy world a great service by producing a book that can sensitise therapists to the sort of issues and dilemmas that problem gamblers face: helping them to create the kind of facilitative environment that will maximise clients' self-explorations. In the fictional examples of Max and Rob, we see two men who experience both the highs and lows of gambling, and two therapists, 'Clive' and 'Pat', who are able to empathise with, and value, both aspects of their being. This is the essence of a person-centred approach – the prizing of *all* of a client – and Richard Bryant-Jefferies shows us here how effectively and sensitively it can be done. As a young man, I would have loved to have had the chance to talk to 'Clive' or 'Pat' and I believe that many other problem gamblers would be helped by such an experience. By bringing such a form of therapeutic relating to the fore, *Counselling for Problem Gamblers* makes a valuable contribution to the psychotherapy and counselling literature.

Mick Cooper PhD
Senior Lecturer in Counselling
University of Strathclyde, Glasgow
May 2005

Preface

In the UK there has been much publicity regarding the idea of introducing super casinos based on American organisations. It has raised questions as to whether this is what people want, with discussions concerning the prevalence of criminality associated with this aspect of the leisure industry. It is also set against the experience of the National Lottery which in 2004 saw its tenth year anniversary and the increasing use of gambling sites on the Internet.

As with any addictive behaviour, the greater the availability, the greater the risk of people becoming addicted to the degree that it has problematic effects on them, and on those closest to them. Many problem gamblers will seek help through counselling and this book aims to demonstrate a person-centred way of working with clients who are seeking to resolve gambling issues.

The success of the preceding books in the *Living Therapy* series, and the continued appreciative comments received from readers and by independent reviewers, is encouragement enough to once again extend this style into exploring the application of the person-centred approach to counselling and psychotherapy to another key area of difficulty within the human experience. Again and again people remark on how readable these books are, how much they bring the therapeutic process alive. In particular, students of counselling and psychotherapy have remarked on how accessible the text is. Trainers and others who are experienced in the field have indicated to me the timeliness of a series that focuses the application of the person-centred approach to working therapeutically with clients having particular issues. This is both heartening and encouraging. I want the style to draw people into the narrative and to make them feel engaged with the characters and the therapeutic process. I want this series to be what I would term 'an experiential read'.

As with the other books in the *Living Therapy* series, *Counselling for Problem Gambling: person-centred dialogues* is composed of fictitious dialogues between fictitious clients and their counsellors, and between their counsellors and their supervisors. Within the dialogues are woven the reflective thoughts and feelings of the clients, the counsellors and the supervisors, along with boxed comments on the process and references to person-centred theory. I do not seek to provide all the answers, or a technical manual expounding on the right way to work with clients who are experiencing a gambling problem. Rather I want to convey something of the process of working with representative material that can arise so that the reader may be stimulated into processing their own reactions, and reflecting on the relevance and effectiveness of the therapeutic responses, to thereby gain insight into themselves and their practice. Often it will simply lead to more questions which I hope will prove stimulating to the reader and encourage them to think through their own theoretical, philosophical and ethical positions and their boundary of competence.

Counselling for Problem Gambling: person-centred dialogues is intended as much for experienced counsellors as it is for trainees. It provides real insight into what can occur during counselling sessions. I hope it will raise awareness of, and inform, not only person-centred practice within this context, but also contribute to other theoretical approaches within the world of counselling, psychotherapy, and the various branches of psychology. Reflections on the therapeutic process and points for discussion are included to stimulate further thought and debate. Included in the book is material to inform the training process of counsellors and others who seek to work with problem gamblers.

This book also has relevance for people who are concerned about their gambling, who may wish to gain an appreciation of a counselling process. It will also serve to inform the gambling industry so that it may be more aware of the processes people may need to undertake in order to resolve gambling problems. It is my hope that this appreciation will encourage the industry to support initiatives to help people who develop problematic gambling habits.

Richard Bryant-Jefferies
May 2005

About the author

Richard Bryant-Jefferies qualified as a person-centred counsellor/therapist in 1994 and remains passionate about the application and effectiveness of this approach. Between early 1995 and mid-2003 Richard worked at a community drug and alcohol service in Surrey as an alcohol counsellor. Since 2003 he has worked for the Central and North West London Mental Health NHS Trust, managing substance misuse service within the Royal Borough of Kensington and Chelsea in London. He has experience of offering counselling and supervision in NHS, GP and private settings, and has provided training through 'alcohol awareness and response' workshops. He also offers workshops based on the use of written dialogue as a contribution to continuing professional development and within training programmes. His website address is www.bryant-jefferies. freeserve.co.uk

Richard had his first book on a counselling theme published in 2001, *Counselling the Person Beyond the Alcohol Problem* (Jessica Kingsley Publishers), providing theoretical yet practical insights into the application of the person-centred approach within the context of the 'cycle of change' model that has been widely adopted to describe the process of change in the field of addiction. Since then he has been writing for the *Living Therapy* series (Radcliffe Publishing), producing an on-going series of person-centred dialogues: *Problem Drinking, Time Limited Therapy in Primary Care, Counselling a Survivor of Child Sexual Abuse, Counselling a Recovering Drug User, Counselling Young People, Counselling for Progressive Disability, Relationship Counselling: sons and their mothers, Responding to a Serious Mental Health Problem, Person-Centred Counselling Supervision: personal and professional, Counselling for Eating Disorders in Men, Counselling for Obesity, Counselling Victims of Warfare* and *Workplace Counselling in the NHS*. The aim of the series is to bring the reader a direct experience of the counselling process, an exposure to the thoughts and feelings of both client and counsellor as they encounter each other on the therapeutic journey, and an insight into the value and importance of supervision.

Richard is also writing his first novel, 'Dying to Live', a story of traumatic loss, alcohol use and the therapeutic and has adapted one of his books as a stage or radio play, and plans to do the same to other books in the series if the first is successful. However, he is currently seeking an opportunity for it to be recorded or staged.

Richard is keen to bring the experience of the therapeutic process, from the standpoint and application of the person-centred approach, to a wider audience.

He is convinced that the principles and attitudinal values of this approach and the emphasis it places on the therapeutic relationship are key to helping people create greater authenticity both in themselves and in their lives, leading to a fuller and more satisfying human experience. By writing fictional accounts to try and bring the therapeutic process alive, to help readers engage with the characters within the narrative – client, counsellor and supervisor – he hopes to take the reader on a journey into the counselling room. Whether we think of it as pulling back the curtains or opening a door, it is about enabling people to access what can and does occur within the therapeutic process.

Acknowledgements

It is with some degree of uncertainty and apprehension that I wait to read what people write by way of their reaction to my books. It is therefore always gratifying to read the encouraging words of those who have a specialist knowledge beyond my own towards a topic that I have addressed. I would like to express my gratitude to both Foreword writers, Professor Mark Griffiths and Mick Cooper. I very much value what they have said, each drawing from their own contrasting involvements with the world of gambling, and yet each conveying a powerful sense of their own relationship to the theme. I could not have asked for more. Thank you to you both.

I would also like to thank GamCare for permission to reproduce pages from its website. Details of how to contact GamCare are included in the Useful contacts section at the end of this book.

I am again indebted to the team at Radcliffe Publishing for its continued commitment to this on-going series of books, and whilst I cannot mention everyone's name, I do wish to thank Maggie Pettifer, Series Editor, and Jamie Etherington who has been very much involved in the production process of all of the *Living Therapy* titles.

Finally, I want to thank my partner, Movena Lucas, for the conversations and the discussions we have had around the theme of gambling, and for being part of my own research process in the amusement arcades at Worthing, Littlehampton and Bognor. I can testify that, yes, those machines do 'pull'. As I heard someone on TV only the other night say in a programme about gambling, 'I could hear the machines calling to me'.

Introduction

Counselling for Problem Gambling: person-centred dialogues demonstrates the application of the person-centred approach (PCA) to counselling and psychotherapy
in working with people who have developed a problematic gambling and betting
habit. This theoretical approach to counselling has, at its heart, the transforming
power of the relational experience.

The PCA is widely used by counsellors working in the UK today: in a member-
ship survey in 2001 by the British Association for Counselling and Psychotherapy, 35.6 per cent of those responding claimed to work to the person-
centred approach, whilst 25.4 per cent identified themselves as psychodynamic
practitioners.

This introduction contains a section on the nature and problem of gambling
and betting, including a focus on adolescent gamblers; an introductory overview
of person-centred theory; an introduction to Rogers' ideas of stages of psychological change; and the use of supervision.

An extended description of the Prochaska and DiClemente (1982) 'cycle of
change' model can be found in the Appendix on page 159. This cycle is widely
used to provide a framework for working with clients with addiction problems in
many addiction services. It provides a more cognitive-behavioural summary of
the stages people pass through in the process of change and whilst it is not a
person-centred model, it has value in extending understanding of the topic.

Gambling and betting

Gambling and taking risks seem to be for many people very much a normalised
way of being. In this book gambling and betting are considered in the context of
putting money in slot-machines, internet gambling, casinos, betting shops and
dog racing; all with the associated element of risk. Other areas not covered are
bingo, the lottery, football and other team sports, and many of the other games
that feature in the casino experience. However, many of the issues are transferable, but not to the point of losing sight of each person's individuality and the
specific reasons for their gambling or betting choices.

Except where a strong religious belief may provide a barrier to establishing a gambling or betting habit, people are affected irrespective of race, social class or economic situation. Some people may be drawn to certain forms of gambling or betting because of their socio-economic situation and that may simply be because of the influence of friends, family and availability. What seems clear is that new forms of betting or gambling, for example via the Internet, have a certain 'trans-socio-economic appeal', and the same might be said of slot-machines where they are situated within casino complexes. Package holidays to Las Vegas will no doubt also have opened up gambling possibilities for people new to that kind of exposure and, of course, there will always be a wide spectrum of people betting on horses – from attendees at Ascot on Ladies' Day to the free-for-all on the hill at the Epsom Derby to visiting the local 'bookies'.

Problem gambling and betting often lead to problems of debt. This is dealt with indirectly in the book. The client with debt problems is referred to a specialist debt counsellor at the Citizen's Advice Bureau (although there are other specialist services available). Some clients will want to talk about their debt problems with their counsellor in relation to their other anxieties.

Gambling

Often 'gambling' and 'betting' seem synonymous but there is a difference. *The Concise Oxford Dictionary* states gambling as, 'Play games of chance for money, esp. for high stakes; take great risks to secure great results in war, finance, etc.'. It also describes gambling as 'a risky undertaking or attempt'. So, risk is involved, but in contrast to betting, gambling is more associated with games of chance. People gamble in the workplace with decisions, with shares, with extra-marital relationships, with other people's lives in hostage situations and in warfare. Some gambles may be 'calculated', but uncertainty remains a significant factor.

In Part 1 of this book the client, Max, who is single, explores his internet gambling habit with his counsellor, Clive. He looks at the origins of his gambling: slot-machines as a child and gaming, and also the impact of his difficult home life and how that contributed to how he internalised his experience in the amusement arcades as something positive, enhancing his sense of self. He explores what those early gambling experiences meant to him and why he continued them. He also looks at the role of Internet gambling in his life; the lure, the attraction to keep gambling, the difficulty in making different choices to fill his time. Internet gambling is an important area of development. It provides widespread availability and a degree of convenience perhaps matched only by the punter watching races on TV and phoning through his bets to the local bookie. However, the twenty-four/seven availability of online gambling provides opportunity for greater problems. Max is offered therapeutic space in which to explore himself, his behaviours and their associations and to affirm within himself his need for change. His formulation of his own strategies to achieve that change is crucially underpinned by his own process of psychological change.

Betting

Betting is, by contrast, less a matter of chance although it does, as with gambling, involve an element of risk. *The Concise Oxford Dictionary* states the word 'bet' means: 'Risk one's money etc., (an amount etc.,) against another's, on the result of a doubtful event (*on* or *against* result or competitor, *that* a thing will happen'. It will therefore be associated with horse and dog racing, football and the many opportunities to wager money on the outcome of sporting events. Not only sport, it could be on election results; anything that involves people and events where uncertainties are present that extend the risk beyond the laws of mathematical probability that tend to be more closely linked to gambling.

In Part 2 of this book, Rob, a married man with a young child, comes into counselling as a result of pressure from his wife. He's had a bad run. He bets regularly at a betting shop but his main betting interest is at the local dog track. It has reached problematic proportions and his attempt to change his habit is complicated by experiencing a win which reinforces his belief that betting is the solution and not the cause of his problems. A couple-session is included when his wife attends counselling because she wants to understand what is happening. Aspects of the couple's relationship are played out within the session. Rob also explores the underlying causes of his betting – they are more associated with conditioning and habit – as attendance at the dog track was an experience learned in childhood with his father. He chooses to work at ways of reducing his betting activity, and in particular managing and reducing it at the betting shop which is also linked to his association with people at work.

When gambling and betting become a problem

When do gambling and betting become a problem? Who needs to experience it as a problem for it to be given this definition? The gambler themselves? Close friends and family? The creditors? The debt counsellor? The debt collector? And what of the gambling industry, at what point might it have a responsibility to draw some-one's attention to their gambling, before it gets further out of control?

In general people begin as 'social gamblers'. It is something they do as part of their lifestyle, giving them a particular set of experiences that are important to them. It satisfies something, whether we call it a need or another name. We do things in order to feel something, often to feel different to the way we felt at the start of whatever it is we are choosing to do. We learn, and we learn fast. 'If I do this, I feel that.' 'If I behave this way, I experience that sensation in myself.' It may be the social context that attracts people to gambling, it may be the lure of the big win, but if you open the door into a betting shop, or you look in on a row of one-arm bandits (one button bandits these days), you will see people who are there to satisfy something in themselves. And part of that may simply be the security that comes from maintaining an habitual behaviour.

Somewhere, though, along the gambling continuum, there is a change from social to problem gambling. It's an invisible line, hard to see it as you approach it, hard to accept it when you're the other side of it. There are indicators that can help people get a sense of whether they have crossed that line: 'Is my gambling causing arguments at home?'. 'Is my gambling something I feel bad about sometimes?' 'Is my gambling something I feel a need to conceal from others?' 'Is my gambling becoming more important in my life, more important than family, work or eating regularly, for example?'

The reality is that this line is crossed when the person's gambling or betting behaviour has a problematic effect on their own lives or that of others, and the gambler persists in the behaviour. The psychological processes behind the decision to gamble, and the gambling choices, will be complex, spanning a range of variables within the human experience.

This book focuses on working with the 'problem gambler' and the 'problem better'; people who have crossed the line and are at various stages in realising that this has happened. It's not easy to accept. And even when someone does, their first response is likely to be to blame others for them being there. People don't set out to be a problem gambler. It happens as a result of various factors that contribute to what may begin as a social experience or an attempt to prove oneself to be a winner, or to be better than the machine, or to simply feel good inside oneself. The problem can begin to dominate part of a person's life to the detriment of the gambler's well-being and that of those around them.

How great is the gambling problem?

Gambling and betting are big business with a high turnover of monies. 'In the UK, the annual turnover, or the amount wagered, on gambling activities is estimated to be in the region of £42 billion. Expenditure or gross gaming yield (amount wagered less winnings paid out) was around £7.3 billion in 1998. Even though casinos have the largest share of turnover (44%), their share of the gross gaming yield is only 6.5% of the total. The National Lottery has the largest share of the gross gaming yield (37%) followed by betting (25%)' (Home Office, 2001).

The popularity of betting is widespread. In terms of which forms of gambling or betting are most popular, the Prevalence Survey shows that within the UK, 65 per cent of people participated in the National Lottery within a given year, 22 per cent gambled with scratchcards, 14 per cent on fruit machines and 13 per cent on betting. This research also shows that more men than women gamble with each form of gambling except when it comes to bingo which is higher amongst women, and scratchcards which are about equal. There is not much difference with regard to the National Lottery, however men are significantly more likely to participate in football pools, horse and dog race betting and table games (Sproston *et al.*, 2000).

The same research indicates that more men than women participate in multiple gambling activities, that twice the number of men as women participated in more than four gambling activities and that more women than men have not gambled.

Young people

Gambling amongst young people and adolescents is an area of increasing concern. It appears that this growing problem is 'related to the high levels of problem gambling generally and other delinquent activities such as illicit drug taking and alcohol abuse' (Griffiths, 2002, p. 5; Griffiths and Sutherland, 1998). Greater availability of gambling opportunities together with increased use of drugs and alcohol affecting judgement and therefore adding to the problematic effect of gambling, are issues that need to be addressed. Research in the 1990s in the UK has indicated that adolescents may be more susceptible to 'pathological gambling' than adults (Griffiths, 2002, p. 4) and references Fisher (1992) as finding that 'among adolescent fruit machine gamblers, 6% did so to a pathological degree'. 'This rate is two or three times higher than that identified in the adult population' (Fisher, 1992; Griffiths, 1995). Sproston *et al.* (2000), for example, found that within the 16 to 24 age band, 1.7 per cent (2.3 per cent men and 1.1 per cent women) were identified as problem gamblers, whilst within the 35 to 44 age band this was 0.8 per cent (2 per cent men and 0.5 per cent women).

There is evidence of strong correlation between adolescent and parental gambling (Griffiths, 1995; Wood and Griffiths, 1998). Also, that gambling in adolescence leads to problematic gambling habits as adults (Fisher 1992; Griffiths 1995). Griffiths has also considered gender in relation to adolescent gambling and finds it to be primarily a male phenomenon (Griffiths, 2002, p. 5; Griffiths, 1991a, b). He also points out that whilst 'there appear to be three main forms of adolescent gambling that have been widely researched (particularly in the UK) – gambling on lotteries, gambling on scratchcards and on fruit machines ... the most problematic appears to be gambling on fruit machines' (Griffiths, 2002, p. 5).

It is difficult to compare studies across the world due to varying age groups, different definitions of gambling and problem gambling, and research design. However, prevalence rates of problem gambling range from 3 per cent in Australia (Moore and Ohtsuka, 1997) to 8.7 per cent in America (Winters *et al.*, 1993).

The research indicates that problem gambling amongst young people needs to be addressed. Our understanding of what draws young people into gambling and of the risk factors that increase the chances of it developing into a problematic habit are becoming better understood as the research continues. As well as the availability and social and economic factors, there is also the need to consider gambling styles and motivational factors that emanate both from within the person and from the design and technology of the fruit and slot-machines that are being considered. Griffiths (2002) comments on these areas, with useful listings of characteristics of adolescent gamblers, risk factors, and practical interventions.

In relation to characteristics Griffiths draws attention to the work of Fisher (1993) who worked part-time at a seaside amusement arcade, and from a sociological perspective undertook non-participant observation supplemented with formal interviews of arcade clientele enabling him to present a typology of amusement arcade players: arcade kings, machine beaters, rent-a-spacers, action seekers and escape artists. He includes lists of characteristics of these five types (Fisher and Bellringer, 1997) and contrasts Fisher's typology with his own research findings (Griffiths, 1991b) from a study from a psychological perspective of participation and non-participation in 33 UK arcades over 28 months. Both present fascinating insights into the types, behaviours and motivations of adolescent fruit machine players with areas of agreement, although Griffiths suggested some groups may be subsets of other groups within the Fisher typology and the reader is encouraged to read these ideas in Griffiths (2002).

Online gambling[1]

- Online gambling is becoming an increasingly popular form of gambling, and there are now an estimated 1700 gambling websites on the Internet and gambling through interactive television and mobile phones is also now possible.
- The convenience of gambling at home, the ease of setting up a gambling account and the variety of forms of gambling – from traditional betting, to casino gambling, bingo and lotteries – makes online gambling very appealing.
- Whilst many people gamble online without any problems, GamCare has started to see an increase in the amount of people contacting its helpline and counselling services because they are losing control of their online gambling.
- The following characteristics of online gambling increase the risk of developing a gambling problem:

  - ability to gamble 24 hours a day in your own home
  - increased risk of exposure and access by children
  - absorption of computers, leading people to lose track of time whilst gambling
  - decrease in the perception of the value of cash – i.e. players are forgetting that they are spending money.

Online tips

- If you are currently gambling online or want to in the future, and are wary of the need to keep control of your gambling, the tips below should help:

  - keep track of the time that you are playing for
  - only spend what you can afford to lose, keep track of your spend whilst playing and remember that the numbers on the screen are REAL MONEY

> – avoid chasing your losses
> – if you're a parent keep your password safe, and if you wish, use software to block access to gambling sites from minors
> – look for sites with options where you can set your own spend and session limits, which should help you to control your gambling
> – if you are having a problem then you can request to be self-excluded from the site. There is also software that blocks access to all online gambling sites. See www.gamblock.com for more details.
>
> [1] Reprinted with the kind permission of GamCare. Website: www.gamcare.org.uk

Conclusion

Gambling and betting are, of course, not problematic for everyone. But where they do reach problematic, addictive or pathological proportions, then the effects can be devastating. The need for appropriate legislation to ensure that gambling is appropriately regulated is required, particularly with gambling and betting now being extended into areas such as the Internet, and the licensing of large casinos in the UK. There is widespread public concern and debate, and rightfully so. In many ways gambling and betting are implicit in human nature, and more so for some people than others. There may be a gambling gene or combination of genes that means individuals are more susceptible to the gambling urge.

Social, familial, economic, demographic and geographic factors can all play a part in contributing to whether a particular person develops a gambling habit and whether it develops into a problematic gambling style. There are also psychological factors to consider – the meaning that a person attributes to their gambling or betting behaviours and experiences, the role it may have in satisfying their physical, emotional and mental needs, which themselves may well be the product of conditioning in early life.

The person seeking to resolve a problem gambling or betting habit will need to feel free to explore themselves, feel that their behaviour is not being judged, that they, as a person, are accepted regardless of the problems they are causing. They will need their unique reasons for their gambling or betting to be understood by the person they are talking to. They will want to feel that the person listening to them is an authentic human-being – not a person who is playing games or manipulating them in some way. And they will probably want to feel that whatever solutions they come up with are their own, that they have contributed to their own process of change rather than feeling something has been imposed upon them which, for many people, may be just the experience that their gambling habit has developed to get them away from. These elements are core features of the person-centred approach that forms the substance of this book. The key features of the person-centred approach to counselling and psychotherapy are described as follows.

The person-centred approach

The person-centred approach (PCA) was formulated by Carl Rogers, and references are made to his ideas within the text of this book. It will be helpful for readers who are unfamiliar with this way of working to have an appreciation of its theoretical base.

Rogers proposed that certain conditions, when present within a therapeutic relationship, would enable the client to develop towards what he termed 'fuller functionality'. Over a number of years he refined these ideas, which he defined as 'the necessary and sufficient conditions for constructive personality change'. These he described as follow.

1   Two persons are in psychological contact.
2   The first, whom we shall term the client, is in a state of incongruence, being vulnerable or anxious.
3   The second person, whom we shall term the therapist, is congruent or integrated in the relationship.
4   The therapist experiences unconditional positive regard for the client.
5   The therapist experiences an empathic understanding of the client's internal frame of reference and endeavours to communicate this experience to the client.
6   The communication to the client of the therapist's empathic understanding and unconditional positive regard is to a minimal degree achieved (Rogers, 1957, p. 96).

The first necessary and sufficient condition given for constructive personality change is that of 'two persons being in psychological contact'. However, although he later published this as simply 'contact' (Rogers, 1959), it is suggested (Wyatt and Sanders, 2002, p. 6) that this was actually written in 1953–4. They quote Rogers as defining contact in the following terms. 'Two persons are in psychological contact, or have the minimum essential relationship when each makes a perceived or subceived difference in the experiential field of the other' (Rogers, 1959, p. 207). A recent exploration of the nature of psychological contact from a person-centred perspective is given by Warner (2002).

Contact

There is much to reflect on when considering a definition of 'contact' or 'psychological contact'. Is contact either present or not? Or is there a continuum, with greater or lesser degrees of contact? It seems to me that it is both. Rather like the way that light may be regarded as either a particle or a wave, contact may be seen as a specific state of being, or as a process, depending upon what the perceiver is seeking to measure or observe. If I am trying to observe or measure whether there is contact, then my answer will be in terms of 'yes' or 'no'. If I am seeking to determine the degree to which contact exists, then the answer will be along a continuum. In other words, from the moment of minimal contact there is contact, but it can extend as more aspects of the client become present within the therapeutic relationship which, itself, may at times reach moments of increasing depth.

Empathy

Rogers defined empathy as meaning 'entering the private perceptual world of the other ... being sensitive, moment by moment, to the changing felt meanings which flow in this other person ... It means sensing meanings of which he or she is scarcely aware, but not trying to uncover totally unconscious feelings' (Rogers, 1980, p. 142). It is a very delicate process, and it provides a foundation block to effective person-centred therapy. The counsellor's role is primarily to establish empathic rapport and communicate empathic understanding to the client. This latter point is vital. Empathic understanding only has therapeutic value where it is communicated to the client.

I would like to add another comment regarding empathy. There is so much more to empathy than simply letting the client know what you understand from what they have communicated. It is also, and perhaps more significantly, the actual *process* of listening to a client, of attending – facial expression, body language, and presence – that is being offered and communicated and received *at the time that the client is speaking, at the time that the client is experiencing what is present for them.* It is, for the client, the knowing that, in the moment of an experience the counsellor is present and striving to be an understanding companion.

Unconditional positive regard

Within the therapeutic relationship the counsellor seeks to maintain an attitude of unconditional positive regard towards the client and all that they disclose. This is not 'agreeing with', it is simply warm acceptance of the fact that the client is being how they need or choose to be. Rogers wrote, 'when the therapist is experiencing a positive, acceptant attitude towards whatever the client *is* at that moment, therapeutic movement or change is more likely to occur' (Rogers, 1980, p. 116). Mearns and Thorne suggest that 'unconditional positive regard is the label given to the fundamental attitude of the person-centred counsellor towards her client. The counsellor who holds this attitude deeply values the humanity of her client and is not deflected in that valuing by any particular client behaviours. The attitude manifests itself in the counsellor's consistent acceptance of and enduring warmth towards her client' (Mearns and Thorne, 1988, p. 59).

Both Bozarth (1998) and Wilkins assert that 'unconditional positive regard is the curative factor in person-centred therapy' (Bozarth and Wilkins, 2001, p. vii). It is perhaps worth speculatively drawing these two statements together. We might then suggest that the unconditional positive regard experienced and conveyed by the counsellor, and received by the client, as an expression of the counsellor's valuing of their client's humanity, has a curative role in the therapeutic process. We might then add that this may be the case more specifically for those individuals who have been affected by a lack of unconditional warmth and prizing in their lives.

Congruence

Last, but by no means least, is that state of being that Rogers referred to as congruence, but which has also been described in terms of 'realness', 'transparency', 'genuineness' and 'authenticity'. Indeed Rogers wrote that '. . . genuineness, realness or congruence . . . this means that the therapist is openly being the feelings and attitudes that are flowing within at the moment. The term transparent catches the flavour of this condition' (Rogers, 1980, p. 115). Putting this into the therapeutic setting, we can say that 'congruence is the state of being of the counsellor when her outward responses to her client consistently match the inner feelings and sensations which she has in relation to her client' (Mearns and Thorne, 1999, p. 84). Interestingly, Rogers makes the following comment in his interview with Richard Evans that with regard to the three conditions: 'first, and most important, is therapist congruence or genuineness . . . one description of what it means to be congruent in a given moment is to be aware of what's going on in your experiencing at that moment, to be acceptant towards that experience, to be able to voice it if it's appropriate, and to express it in some behavioural way' (Evans, 1975).

I would suggest that any congruent expression by the counsellor of their feelings or reactions has to emerge through the process of being in therapeutic relationship with the client. Indeed, the condition indicates that the therapist is congruent or integrated into the relationship. This indicates the significance of the relationship. Being congruent is a disciplined way of being and not an open door to endless self-disclosure. Congruent expression is perhaps most appropriate and therapeutically valuable where it is informed by the existence of an empathic understanding of the client's inner world, and is offered in a climate of a genuine warm acceptance towards the client. Having said that, it is reasonable to suggest that, taking Rogers' comment quoted above regarding congruence as 'most important', we might suggest that unless the therapist is congruent in themselves and in the relationship, then their empathy and unconditional positive regard would be at risk of not being authentic or genuine.

Another view, however, would be that it is in some way false to distinguish or rather seek to separate the three 'core conditions'; rather they exist together as a whole, mutually dependent on each other in order to ensure that therapeutic relationship is established.

Perception

There is also the sixth condition, of which Rogers wrote: 'the final condition ... is that the client perceives, to a minimal degree, the acceptance and empathy which the therapist experiences for him. Unless some communication of these attitudes has been achieved, then such attitudes do not exist in the relationship as far as the client is concerned, and the therapeutic process could not, by our hypothesis, be initiated' (Rogers, 1957). It is interesting that he uses the words 'minimal degree', suggesting that the client does not need to fully perceive the fullness of the empathy and unconditional positive regard present within, and communicated by, the counsellor. A glimpse accurately heard and empathically understood is enough to have positive, therapeutic effect although logically one might think that the more that is perceived, the greater the therapeutic impact. But if it is a matter of intensity and accuracy, then a client experiencing a vitally important fragment of their inner world being empathically understood may be more significant to them, and more therapeutically significant, than a great deal being heard less accurately and with a weaker sense of therapist understanding. The communication of the counsellor's empathy, congruence and unconditional positive regard, received by the client, creates the conditions for a process of constructive personality change.

Relationship is key

The PCA regards the relationship that counsellors have with their clients, and the attitude that they hold within that relationship, to be key factors. In my experience, many adult psychological difficulties develop out of life experiences that involve problematic, conditional or abusive relational experiences. This can be centred in childhood or later in life, and in this book we focus on the development of gambling and betting habits which, themselves, become problematic. What is significant is that the individual is left, through relationships that have a negative conditioning effect, with a distorted perception of themselves and their potential as a person. Patterns are established in early life, bringing their own particular problems, however they can be exacerbated by conditional and psychologically damaging experiences later in life, that in some cases will have a resonance to what has occurred in the past, exacerbating the effects still further.

An oppressive experience can impact on a child's confidence in themselves, leaving them anxious, uncertain and moving towards establishing patterns of thought, feeling and behaviour associated with the developing concept of themselves typified by 'I am weak and cannot expect to be treated any differently' and 'I just have to accept this attitude towards me, what can I do to change anything?'. These psychological conclusions may rest on patterns of thinking and feeling already established, perhaps the person was bullied at school, or experienced rejection in the home. They may have had a life-time of stress, or it may be a relatively new experience; either way they may develop a way of thinking typified by 'it's normal to feel stressed, you just keep going, whatever it takes'.

The result is a conditioned sense of self, with the individual then thinking, feeling and acting in ways that enable them to maintain their self-beliefs and meanings within their learned or adapted concept of self. This is then lived out, the person seeking to satisfy what they have come to believe about themselves: needing to care either because it has been normalised, or in order to prove to themselves and the world that they are a 'good' person. They will need to maintain this conditioned sense of self and the sense of satisfaction that this gives them when it is lived out because they have developed such a strong identity with it. A gambling or betting habit can be one factor in maintaining a particular sense of self, or in creating a new one in order to escape from discomfort.

The term 'conditions of worth', applies to the conditioning mentioned previously that is frequently present in childhood, and at other times in life, when a person experiences that their worth is conditional on their doing something, or behaving, in a certain way. This is usually to satisfy someone else's needs, and can be contrary to the client's own sense of what would be a satisfying experience. The values of others become a feature of the individual's structure of self. The person moves away from being true to themselves, learning instead to remain 'true' to their conditioned sense of worth. This state of being in the client is challenged by the person-centred therapist by offering them unconditional positive regard and warm acceptance. Such a therapist, by genuinely offering these therapeutic attitudes, provides the client with an opportunity to be exposed to what may be a new experience or one that in the past they have dismissed, preferring to stay with that which matches and therefore reinforces their conditioned sense of worth and sense of self.

By offering someone a non-judgemental, warm and accepting, and authentic relationship, (perhaps a kind of 'therapeutic love'?), that person can grow into a fresh sense of self in which their potential as a person can become more fulfilled. It enables them to liberate themselves from the constraints of patterns of conditioning. Such an experience fosters an opportunity for the client to redefine themselves as they experience the presence of the therapist's congruence, empathy and unconditional positive regard. This process can take time. Often the personality change that is required to sustain a shift away from what have been termed 'conditions of worth' may require a lengthy period of therapeutic work, bearing in mind that the person may be struggling to unravel a sense of self that has been developed, sustained and reinforced over many decades of life. Of course, where the sense of self has been established more recently then less time may be necessary.

Actualising tendency

A crucial feature or factor in this process of 'constructive personality change' is the presence of what Rogers termed 'the actualising tendency', a tendency towards fuller and more complete personhood with an associated greater fulfilment of their potentialities. The role of the person-centred counsellor is to provide the facilitative climate within which this tendency can work constructively. The 'therapist trusts the actualizing tendency of the client and truly believes that the client who experiences the freedom of a fostering psychological climate will resolve his or her own problems' (Bozarth, 1998, p. 4). This is fundamental to the application of the person-centred approach. Rogers (1986, p. 198) wrote: 'the person-centred approach is built on a basic trust in the person ... [It] depends on the actualizing tendency present in every living organism – the tendency to grow, to develop, to realize its full potential. This way of being trusts the constructive directional flow of the human being towards a more complex and complete development. It is this directional flow that we aim to release'.

Having said the above, we must also acknowledge that for some people, or at certain stages, rather than producing a liberating experience, there will instead be a tendency to maintain the status quo, perhaps the fear of change, the uncertainty, or the implications of change are such that the person prefers to maintain the known, the certain. In a sense, there is a liberation from the imperative to change and grow which may bring temporary – and perhaps permanent – relief for the person. The actualising tendency may work through the part of the person that needs relief from change, enhancing its presence for the period of time that the person experiences a need to maintain this. The person-centred therapist will not try to move the person from this place or state. It is to be accepted, warmly and unconditionally. And, of course, sometimes in the moment of acceptance the person is enabled to question whether that really is how they want to be.

Configuration within self

It is of value to draw attention, at this point, to the notion of 'configurations within self'. Configurations within self (Mearns and Thorne, 2000) are discrete sets of thoughts, feelings and behaviours that develop through the experience of life. They emerge in response to a range of experiences including the process of introjection and the symbolisation of experiences, as well as in response to dissonant self-experience within the person's structure of self. They can also exist in what Mearns terms as '"growthful" and "not for growth", configurations' (Mearns and Thorne, 2000, pp. 114–6), each offering a focus for the actualising tendency, the former seeking an expansion into new areas of experience with all that that brings, the latter seeking to energise the status quo and to block change because of its potential for disrupting the current order within the structure of self. The actualising tendency may not always manifest through growth or developmental change. It can also manifest through periods of stabilisation and stability, or a wanting to get away from something. The self, then, is seen as a constellation of configurations with the individual moving between them and living through them in response to experience.

Mearns suggests that these 'parts' or 'configurations' interrelate 'like a family, with an individual variety of dynamics'. As within any 'system', change in one area will impact on the functioning of the system. He therefore comments that 'when the interrelationship of configurations changes, it is not that we are left with something entirely new: we have the same "parts" as before, but some which may have been subservient before are stronger, others which were judged adversely are accepted, some which were in self-negating conflict have come to respect each other, and overall the parts have achieved constructive integration with the energy release which arises from such fusion' (Mearns and Thorne, 1999, pp. 147–8). The growing acceptance of the configurations, their own fluidity and movement within the self-structure, the increased, open and more accurate communication between the parts, is, perhaps, another way of considering the integrating of the threads of experience to which Rogers refers.

In terms of these ideas, we can anticipate clients containing, within themselves, particular configurations with which certain gambling behaviours are associated. So, a configuration may have developed that associates a gambling behaviour with feeling in control in an uncertain world, or with experiencing the release of adrenaline to give the person a feeling of strength and excitement. Or perhaps a dominant 'gambling configuration' may develop that contains the many thoughts, feelings and behaviours associated with that person's gambling pattern, a part of that person's structure of self that assumes a certain psychological primacy which, in turn, means the associated gambling behaviour then also takes a similar position in the person's life. There may also be 'not for gambling' configurations as well, or these may emerge through the process of working at dealing with the issues in therapy. Understanding the configurational nature of ourselves enables us to understand why we are triggered into certain thoughts, feelings and behaviours, and how they group together, serving a particular experiential purpose for the person.

From this theoretical perspective we can argue that the person-centred counsellor's role is essentially facilitative. Creating the therapeutic climate of empathic understanding, unconditional positive regard and authenticity creates a relational climate which encourages the client to move into a more fluid state with more openness to their own experience and the discovery of a capacity towards a fuller actualising of their potential.

Relationship re-emphasised

In addressing these factors the therapeutic relationship is central. A therapeutic approach such as the person-centred one affirms that it is not what you do so much as *how you are* with your client that is therapeutically significant, and this 'how you are' has to be received by the client. Gaylin (2001, p. 103) highlights the importance of client perception. 'If clients believe that their therapist is working on their behalf – if they perceive caring and understanding – then therapy is likely to be successful. It is the condition of attachment and the perception of connection that have the power to release the faltered actualization of the self.' He goes on to stress how 'we all need to feel connected, prized – loved', describing human-beings as 'a species born into mutual interdependence', and that there 'can be no self outside the context of others. Loneliness is dehumanizing, and isolation anathema to the human condition. The relationship,' he suggests 'is what psychotherapy is all about.'

Love is an important word though not necessarily one often used to describe therapeutic relationship. Patterson, however, gives a valuable definition of love as it applies to the person-centred therapeutic process. He writes, 'we define love as an attitude that is expressed through empathic understanding, respect and compassion, acceptance, and therapeutic genuineness, or honesty and openness towards others' (Patterson, 2000, p. 315). We all need love, but most of all we need it during our developmental period of life. The same author affirms that 'whilst love is important throughout life for the well-being of the individual, it is particularly important, indeed absolutely necessary, for the survival of the infant and for providing the basis for the normal psychological development of the individual' (Patterson, 2000, pp. 314–5).

In a previous book in this series I used the analogy of treating a wilting plant (Bryant-Jefferies, 2003, p. 12). We can spray it with a herbicide or pesticide to eradicate a perceived disease that may be present in the plant, and that may be enough. But perhaps the true cause of the disease is that the plant is located in harsh surroundings, perhaps too much sun and not enough water, poor soil, near other plants that it finds difficulty in surviving so close to. Maybe by offering the plant a healthier environment that will facilitate greater nourishment according to its needs will lead to it becoming the strong, healthy plant it has the potential to be. Yes, the chemical intervention may also be helpful, but if the true causes of the disease are environmental – essentially the plant's relationship with that which surrounds it – then it won't actually achieve sustainable growth. We may not be able to transplant it, but we can provide water, nutrients and maybe shade from a fierce sun. Therapy, it seems to me, exists to provide this healthy environment within which the 'wilting' client can begin the process of receiving the nourishment (in the form of healthy relational experience) that can enable them, in time, to become a more fully functioning person.

Process of change from a person-centred perspective

Rogers was interested in understanding the process of change, what it was like, how it occurred and what experiences it brought to those involved – client and therapist. At different points he explored this. Embleton Tudor *et al.* (2004) point to a model consisting of 12 steps identified in 1942 (Rogers, 1942) and to Rogers' two later chapters on this topic (Rogers, 1951), and finally the seven-stage model (Rogers, 1967). He wrote of 'initially looking for elements which would mark or characterize change itself', however, what he experienced from his enquiry and research into the process of change he summarised as: 'individuals move, I began to see, not from fixity or homeostasis through change to a new fixity, though such a process is indeed possible. But much the more significant continuum is from fixity to changingness, from rigid structure to flow, from stasis to process. I formed the tentative hypothesis that perhaps the qualities of the client's expression at any one point might indicate his position on this continuum, where he stood in the process of change' (Rogers, 1967).

Change, then, involves a movement from fixity to greater fluidity, from, we might say, a rigid set of attitudes and behaviours to a greater openness to experience, to variety and diversity. Change might be seen as having a certain liberating quality, a freeing up of the human-being – his heart, mind, emotions – so that the person experiences themselves less of a fixed object and more of a conscious process. For the client who is seeking to resolve issues associated with problematic gambling, part of this process will involve a loosening of the individual's identity as being strongly connected to the image they have of themselves as a gambler and addressing the psychological experiencing that flows from the gambling experience. Until this is 'unfixed', if you like, it would seem reasonable to conclude that sustained controlled gambling or abstinence might be extremely difficult to achieve.

The list below is taken from Rogers' summary of the process, indicating the changes that people will show.

1   This process involves a loosening of feelings.
2   This process involves a change in the manner of experiencing.
3   The process involves a shift from incongruence to congruence.
4   The process involves a change in the manner in which, and the extent to which the individual is able and willing to communicate himself in a receptive climate.
5   The process involves a loosening of the cognitive maps of experience.
6   There is a change in the individual's relationship to his problem.
7   There is a change in the individual's manner of relating (Rogers, 1967, pp. 156–8).

This is a very brief overview, the chapter in which Rogers describes the process of change has much more detail and should be read in order to gain a clear grasp not only of the process as a whole, but of the distinctive features of each stage, as he saw it. Embleton Tudor *et al.* summarise this process in the following, and I think helpful, terms: 'a movement from fixity to fluidity, from closed to open, from tight to loose, and from afraid to accepting' (2004, p. 47).

In Rogers' description of the process he makes the point that there were several types of process by which personality changes and that the process he described is one that is 'set in motion when the individual experiences himself as being fully received'. Does this process apply to all psychotherapies? Rogers indicated that more data were needed, adding that 'perhaps therapeutic approaches which place great stress on the cognitive and little on the emotional aspects of experience may set in motion an entirely different process of change'. In terms of whether this process of change would generally be viewed as desirable and that it would move the person in a valued direction, Rogers expressed the view that the valuing of a particular process of change was linked to social value judgements made by individuals and cultures. He pointed out that the process of change that he described could be avoided, simply by people 'reducing or avoiding those relationships in which the individual is fully received as he is' (Rogers, 1967).

Rogers also took the view that change was unlikely to be rapid, making the point that many clients enter the therapeutic process at stage two, and leave at stage four, having during that period gained enough to feel satisfied. He suggested it would be 'very rare, if ever, that a client who fully exemplified stage one would move to a point where he fully exemplified stage seven', and that if this did occur 'it would involve a matter of years' (Rogers, 1967, pp. 155–6). He wrote of how, at the outset, the threads of experience are discerned and understood separately by the client but as the process of change takes place, they move into 'the flowing peak moments of therapy in which all these threads become inseparably woven together.' He continues: 'in the new experiencing with immediacy which occurs at such moments, feeling and cognition interpenetrate, self is subjectively present in the experience, volition is simply the subjective following of a harmonious balance of organismic direction. Thus, as the process reaches this point the person becomes a unity of flow, of motion. He has changed, but what seems most significant, he has become an integrated process of changingness' (Rogers, 1967, p. 158).

It conjures up images of flowing movement, perhaps we should say purposeful flowing movement as being the essence of the human condition; a state that we each have the potential to become, or to realise. Is it something we generate or develop out of fixity, or does it exist within us all as a potential that we lose during our conditional experiencing in childhood? Are we discovering something new, or re-discovering something that was lost?

In the context of this book, we need to consider an holistic approach, with both gambling behaviours and psychological processes inter-relating (as they do) within the therapeutic process. Each will contribute to, and inform, the other process, a kind of feedback loop being generated; the system evolving and developing by feeding off the changes made and the experiences that those changes bring into awareness. The more satisfying to the person the experience of change is, the greater their motivation will be to pursue change further. In this process of psychological change, the re-balancing and integrating process then becomes evidenced through changes in gambling behaviour.

Supervision

Supervision sessions are included in the book to offer the reader insight into the nature of therapeutic supervision in the context of the counselling profession, a method of supervising that I term 'collaborative review'. For many trainee counsellors, the use of supervision can be something of a mystery, and it is hoped that this book will go a long way to unravelling this. In the supervision sessions I seek to demonstrate the application of the supervisory relationship. My intention is to show how supervision of the counsellor is very much a part of the process of enabling a client to work through issues that in this case relate to traumatic events linked to gambling.

Many professions do not recognise the need for some form of personal and process supervision, and often what is offered is line-management. However, counsellors are required to receive regular supervision in order to explore the dynamics of the relationship with a client, the impact of the work on the counsellor and on the client, to receive support, to encourage professional development of the counsellor and to provide an opportunity for an experienced co-professional to monitor the supervisee's work in relation to ethical standards and codes of practice. The supervision sessions are included because they are an integral part of the therapeutic process. It is also hoped that they will help readers from other professions to recognise the value of some form of supportive and collaborative supervision in order to help them become more authentically present with their own clients.

Merry describes what he termed as 'collaborative inquiry' as a 'form of research or inquiry in which two people (the supervisor and the counsellor) collaborate or co-operate in an effort to understand what is going on within the counselling relationship and within the counsellor'. He emphasises how this 'moves the emphasis away from "doing things right or wrong" (which seems to be the case in some approaches to supervision) to "how is the counsellor being, and how is that way of being contributing to the development of the counselling relationship based on the core conditions" ' (Merry, 2002, p. 173). Elsewhere, Merry describes the relationship between person-centred supervision and congruence, indicating that 'a state of congruence … is the necessary condition for the therapist to experience empathic understanding and unconditional positive regard' (Merry, 2001, p. 183). Effective person-centred supervision provides a means through which congruence can be promoted within the therapist.

Tudor and Worrall (2004) have drawn together a number of theoretical and experiential strands from within and outside of the person-centred tradition in order to develop a theoretical position on the person-centred approach to supervision. In my view, this is a timely publication, defining the necessary factors for effective supervision within this way of working, and the respective responsibilities of both supervisor and supervisee in keeping with person-centred values and principles. They contrast person-centred working with other approaches to supervision and emphasise the importance of the therapeutic space as a place within which practitioners 'can dialogue freely between their personal philosophy and the philosophical assumptions which underlie their chosen theoretical orientation' (Tudor and Worrall, 2004, pp. 94–5). They affirm the values and attitudes of person-centred working and explore their application to the supervisory relationship.

In my own writing (Bryant-Jefferies, 2005) I have sought to demonstrate the process of person-centred supervision in relation to a range of issues drawn from the *Living Therapy* series.

There are, of course, as many models of supervision as there are models of counselling. In this book the supervisor is seeking to apply the attitudinal qualities of the person-centred approach.

It is the norm for all professionals working in the healthcare and social care environment in this age of regulation to be formally accredited or registered and to work to their own professional organisation's code of ethics or practice. For instance, registered counselling practitioners with the British Association for Counselling and Psychotherapy are required to have regular supervision and continuing professional development to maintain registration. Whilst professions other than counsellors will gain much from this book in their work, it is essential that they follow the standards, safeguards and ethical codes of their own professional organisation, and are appropriately trained and supervised to work with them on the issues that arise.

Dialogue format

The reader who has not read other titles in the *Living Therapy* series may find it takes a while to adjust to the dialogue format. Many of the responses offered by the counsellors, Clive and Pat, are reflections of what their respective clients, Max and Rob, have said. This is not to be read as conveying a simple repetition of the clients' words. Rather, the counsellor seeks to voice empathic responses, often with a sense of 'checking out' that they are hearing accurately what the client is saying. The client says something; the counsellor then conveys what they have heard, what they sense the client as having sought to communicate to them, sometimes with the same words, sometimes with words that include a sense of what they feel is being communicated through the client's tone of voice, facial expression, or simply the relational atmosphere of the moment. The client is then enabled to confirm that she has been heard accurately, or correct the counsellor in her perception. The client may then explore more deeply what they have been saying or move on, in either case with a sense that they have been heard and warmly accepted. To draw this to the reader's attention, I have included some of the inner thoughts and feelings that are present within the individuals who form the narrative.

The sessions are a little compressed. It is also fair to say that clients will take different periods of time before choosing to disclose particular issues, and will also take varying lengths of time in working with their own process. This book is not intended to in any way indicate the length of time that may be needed to work with the kinds of issues that are being addressed. The counsellor needs to be open and flexible to the needs of the client. For some clients, the process may take a lot longer. But there are also clients who are ready to talk about difficult experiences almost immediately – sometimes not feeling that they have much choice in the matter as their own organismic processes are already driving memories, feelings, thoughts and experiences to the surface and into daily awareness.

All characters in this book are fictitious and are not intended to bear resemblance to any particular person or persons. These fictional accounts are not aimed at trying to encompass all possible causes of problem gambling, they simply highlight some of the behavioural, emotional, cognitive, psychological and social factors that can be associated for some people. Others will have developed a problem gambling habit for other reasons, however, the response from the person-centred approach will be similar to that described in this book.

I am extremely encouraged by the increasing interest in the person-centred approach, the growing amount of material being published, and the realisation that relationship is a key factor in positive therapeutic outcome. There is currently much debate about theoretical developments within the person-centred world and its application. Discussions on the theme of Rogers' therapeutic conditions presented by various key members of the person-centred community have recently been published (Bozarth and Wilkins, 2001; Haugh and Merry, 2001; Wyatt, 2001; Wyatt and Sanders, 2002). Mearns and Thorne have produced a timely publication revising and developing key aspects of person-centred theory (2000). Wilkins has produced a book that addresses most effectively many of the criticisms levelled against person-centred working (Wilkins, 2003) and Embleton Tudor *et al.* (2004) an introduction to the person-centred approach that places the theory and practice within a contemporary context.

Recently, Howard Kirschenbaum (Carl Rogers' biographer) published an article entitled 'The current status of Carl Rogers and the person-centered approach'. In his research for this article he noted that from 1946–86, 84 books, 64 chapters, and 456 journal articles were published on Carl Rogers and the PCA. In contrast, from 1987–2004 there were 141 books, 174 book chapters and 462 journal articles published. These data show a clear trend towards more publications and, presumably more readership and interest in the approach. Also, he observed that there are now 50 person-centred publications available around the world, mostly journals, and there are now person-centred organisations in 18 countries, and 20 organisations overall. He also draws attention to the large body of research demonstrating the effectiveness of person-centred therapy, concluding that the person-centred approach is 'alive and well' and appears to be experiencing 'something of a revival, both in professional activity and academic respectability' (Kirschenbaum, 2005).

This is obviously a very brief introduction to the PCA. Person-centred theory continues to develop as practitioners and theoreticians consider its application in various fields of therapeutic work and extend our theoretical understanding of developmental and therapeutic processes. At times it feels like it has become more than just individuals, rather it feels like a group of colleagues, based around the world, working together to penetrate deeper towards a more complete theory of the human condition, and this includes people from the many psychotherapeutic traditions and schools of thought. Person-centred or client-centred theory and practice has a key role in this process. Theories are being re-visited and developed, new ideas speculated upon, new media explored for presenting the core values and philosophy of the PCA. It is an exciting time.

PART I

The gambling habit

CHAPTER I

Counselling session 1: the client introduces his gambling

Max sat in the waiting area, feeling anxious in the chair. He looked around him. It seemed quite busy. An elderly woman was sitting opposite, she was wearing a beige coat and had white hair. She was looking down at her hands in her lap. She hadn't moved much since he had sat down himself. Next to her was a rather overweight man with a bald head who looked like he drank a lot judging by the shape of his stomach. A young woman, very thin, was to his left, with a pram next to her. The baby in the pram was very quiet. To his right, there was a man reading a magazine, looking quite relaxed. No one was speaking. Max had come to see a counsellor about his gambling and he wondered what problems the other people had who were waiting.

On the wall was a sign, "psychological therapies". Max thought about the circumstances that had led to him being there. It was a long story. He guessed he'd have to go through it with the person he was seeing – Clive was his name. They'd spoken on the phone and, well, he'd seemed OK. Clive hadn't asked too many questions, he was more concerned with what Max wanted from counselling rather than what had happened to him in the past. It wasn't quite what he'd expected. What was it that Clive had said? Oh yes, "so, you feel trapped by something that makes you feel so good?" It was after he'd made some comment himself about how he felt unable to change his gambling habit, something that he actually didn't want to change, at least, he didn't want to lose the feeling that it gave him, and not just the feeling, but the lifestyle, the friends, the atmosphere, the exhilaration, everything that came with it.

A man came into the waiting area, the first thing that Max noted was his black face. It wasn't that he had any problems with it, but somehow he was surprised. For some reason he'd made an assumption that the staff would be white. He wasn't sure why, it was just what he had thought. Maybe it was the area he lived in – mainly white, although he had friends from other racial backgrounds. He heard the man say his name.

'Yes, that's me.' And he made to get up.

'Hi, I'm Clive, we spoke on the phone.' The man was offering his hand as Max walked towards him. 'Hi, I'm Max.'

Clive nodded. 'Follow me. Can I get you a tea or coffee or anything?'

'No, no thanks. I'm fine.'

'OK. Well, come on through.' Clive walked into the counselling room and Max followed.

'Have a seat.'

'Max looked at the two chairs and looked back to Clive, looking for a clue as to which one he should sit in.'

'Either one, up to you.'

Max moved towards the chair on the left, it was slightly closer and was sort of in the direction he had been heading in as he had come through the door. He took off his jacket, hung it over the back of the seat and sat down.

'So, we talked on the phone about what you were hoping to gain from counselling, and I explained about confidentiality, and we sent you the leaflet as well, yes?'

Max nodded.

'Do you have any questions, is there anything you are unsure about?'

Max shook his head.

'And is the chair comfortable, and do you feel OK with them arranged like this?'

Max nodded. He had felt a little unsure about what was going to happen, but he felt OK about being there. He'd had counselling before and it hadn't really helped very much. But then, well, at the time he hadn't really wanted to change. He'd talked about his gambling but the counsellor seemed more intent on trying to make him accept he had to stop. He didn't think so, he felt sure he could control the situation. He'd only gone because they'd had some financial problems. He'd mentioned it to Clive, and Clive had told him that it sounded as though he'd seen more of a financial advisor or a debt advisor – it had been at the Citizen's Advice Bureau – rather than a therapeutic counsellor. Clive had explained the difference and he sort of understood.

Max had been referred this time by his GP. He'd been feeling depressed – things hadn't been going too well, bit of an unlucky run – it happened. But it had caused problems at home and, well, to keep the peace he'd mentioned it to his doctor when he was seeing him because of his low mood and difficulty in getting himself out to work. He was a manager in an advertising company, quite a creative job, and it was well paid. That was part of the problem. He'd never really been able to hang on to money, right from being a teenager. Down the arcade on the pier, that was where it had all started, with his mates. Somewhere to go, something to do. Never seemed a problem. No, never had seemed a problem, it was what they all did. Had to have a bit of fun and, yeah … He smiled as he thought back to those days. Crazy days.

Clive noticed Max smiling. 'You looked a bit lost in thought there, and it seemed to make you smile.'

'Hmm? Oh, yes, yes, thinking about the past.'

'About the past?'

'Yes, well, back to when it started.'

'Mhmm, back to when it started.'

'Seems a long time ago and yet it doesn't as well.' He shook his head. 'You know, my life has been a series of different gambling experiences. Yes, there have been other things as well, but it's been quite a feature and, well, it kind of grows on you. It's not a problem, until suddenly it is, and you're owing money, but you think the next bet will be the one, it's always the next bet. And sometimes, yes, sometimes it is, and you do win. But often you don't, but then again it's the same thought, OK, I was unlucky, and you find something to blame. The way the cards were shuffled, maybe, but you know next time it'll be OK. You have to win, you have to. It's a drug, man, it really is.' Max shook his head again. 'But you don't see it. Just started out having a few laughs with my mates. Just that.'

'That's how it started out, a few laughs with your mates.'

The counsellor empathises with the end of what the client has said by staying with the flow and not pulling the client's focus back over what he has said but in his own process has moved on from. Sometimes a summarising empathic response can have value, at other times it is best to stay with where the client has reached to enable them to continue with their own flow of thoughts, feelings and experiencing.

Max nodded. 'We'd head off after school, and later when we should have been at school as well. Bunk off down to the arcades. Sometimes we'd be on the games to win money, but not always. The driving games, they'd be a real attraction too. Grand prix, rallying, whatever. It was a buzz. And the fighting games.' He paused. 'In a way playing to win money wasn't the first motivation, it was to have a laugh, have fun, get a buzz, you know? We'd mess around, yeah, and get thrown out sometimes. But we'd go elsewhere – there were a lot of places to choose between living by the sea, you know? Place was all bright lights and stuff.'

Clive nodded. He could sense the allure. 'Yes, somewhere to go, feel drawn to, and it gave you a buzz.'

'It did, and, well, we'd have our pocket money, and we all did a few jobs to earn a bit more, always ways to get a bit of money, you know? That's how it was.' Max was also aware that it was later that they'd got into robbing, not much, but a little now and then, stuff they'd then sell on. Usually things they'd lifted from market stalls. They'd also found they could get money from begging as well, or claiming they hadn't got a fare to get home. That used to work too.

'Mhmm, you'd always be able to get some money.'

'So, yeah, we'd be down the arcades, messing around. Never thought it would become a problem. I mean, it wasn't, you know?'

'No reason to experience it as a problem then?'

Max shook his head. 'And it never has really felt a problem, not really. Even when things were bad and the debts were mounting up, it still wasn't a problem, not in my head. Gambling was never a problem, and I can still feel that it doesn't seem like a problem, even now, although I know it is as well.'

'So you know it's a problem now but it doesn't feel like a problem, and never has?'

Max thought about it. That did sound how it was. 'Yeah, weird that. It's always been a solution, not a problem. It's what I've always done to sort out my money situation, I suppose. Although not to begin with. No, that was something later. Began to be part of it, to gamble, bet, whatever, to make up for what I'd lost, what I'd owed. But to begin with, it was the buzz, felt good, and the boost from winning.' Max shook his head. 'Yeah, winning . . . And that's still there.'

'The urge to win, to re-live that experience again, you mean?'

'Only now it's different, it's more intense.'

'What you do now is more intense?'

Max nodded. 'It's the Internet that did it for me. Twenty-four/seven gambling. To begin with, yeah, that felt exactly what I needed, but . . .' He sighed heavily. 'You just keep going, and, well, when you reach your limit on one credit card, you use another, and another, and so it goes on. You don't care, why should you? You don't want to think about it. You ignore the statements. They don't do anything to make you pay, so the numbers keep going up, but so what? You can't pay it anyway. Maybe you'll get the big win, maybe, but actually you're not thinking about what you owe. It's still about winning, beating the system, beating the machine, that's what it is for me. I have to feel I can win, gives me a good feeling.'

'That feeling, sounds as though it's a real drive for you in gambling?'

Max nodded again. 'For me, yes. Maybe different for others, but for me, it's about feeling . . .' He paused, thinking about how best it was to describe how it felt. 'There's an exhilaration, you feel big, expanded, you feel yourself smiling. You've beaten whatever, whoever, and it feels great. It really does. It . . . I don't know, and then you're wanting it again. There's the next deal and away you go again. Always chasing that feeling, chasing that excitement. And part of it is there during the game, the hope, the expectation, you're on the edge. You're focused as well, yes, there's something about that too. You're focused, you're clear, everything else drops away. All that matters is the next card. It becomes your whole world. Everything becomes that next card. It's tense and the tension, it's really . . .' Max was nodding as he spoke, '. . . really important as well.'

'So chasing that feeling, the excitement, the exhilaration, feeling the tension as you wait for the next card.'

'Knowing you are going to win, you have to win, it's your right to win. All these thoughts. You know it's your turn to win, you know it.' He sniffed, and raised his hands slightly before dropping them into his lap. 'And then it's the wrong card, you grit your teeth. It wasn't your fault. You did the right thing. You stayed with what you had, you were unlucky. The cards, they were against you, but next time, immediately, next time . . .' Another pause. 'And so it goes on. And, yeah, I've had winning streaks, and sometimes I've held on to it, but usually I've lost it. Why can't you stop when you are ahead? But it's so fucking difficult.'

'Sounds like that's what you wish you could do, stop when you're ahead?'

'But you rarely do. At least, that's how it is for me.'

'Mhmm, rarely able to stop when you're ahead.'

'Except if I had to. It's like when you're losing you keep going in the hope of cutting your losses, you know? But if you've won and then start losing, you've got to get your money back. It's your money they've now got. And I still get caught up by it. I still can't stop even though I know I have to, but it's compelling, but I have to stop. That's why I'm here.'

'So, you've realised you have to stop?'

'I've known it for a while, and, well, I'm trying to but I don't know, it's too easy to keep going . . . I need some ideas.'

'So, some new ideas for making changes?'

'And as I've been speaking just now, I can see it is an addiction, I know that, and I know it's going to get me nowhere, but it's so much a part of me, of who I am, what I do. I mean, I'm not a professional gambler, I work, you know, but I can spend so much time being pulled into it.'

'So you spend a lot of your time gambling?'

The client has said very little about his current gambling practice, he is more focused on the past, on how it started. The person-centred counsellor will not be imposing a formal history-taking on the client, but instead will allow the picture to develop as the client communicates whatever he or she wants the counsellor to know. The client, in being allowed a free rein to go with his own flow, will be experiencing himself in a relational climate that encourages freedom. The client's train of thought and feeling may well jump around, at least that is how it might seem from the outside, but for the client there will be links and associations. Being allowed to tell it in his own way, at his own pace, is an important feature of person-centred counselling. Invariably, the information that might have been obtained from a formal assessment will arise. In a very real sense, it is an on-going process, and in many ways becomes as much a self-assessment, an opportunity for the client to assess their situation, themselves, their experiences, as anything else.

This process of self-assessment is an important aspect of the person-centred way of working with a client. The counsellor does not know what are the key elements. Often assessments are factual – about places, people and events, and follow a set series of questions or topics. But in a non-directive self-assessment process the client is not only recalling events, but is also engaging with a flow of thoughts and feelings emerging from within themselves. If, as the person-centred approach argues, the client's internal process is essentially trustworthy, if the client is the person who knows best what they need to focus on, then formal, structured assessments can limit the scope for the client to feel and experience their own flow of meaning in association with the events that they recall. The assessment process is, or

> should be, part of the therapeutic process. For this to be so, it has to be experienced as therapeutic. The following principles of person-centred practice therefore need to be applied: non-directiveness, empathic responding, warm acceptance and congruence.

Max nodded. 'Too much, I know that.'

'So, you know it's too much.'

'Time and money. Funny, never been a sporting gambler. Don't know why. Never felt drawn to the horses, that kind of thing. But cards, yeah, that's the one for me these days, and sometimes I'll also bet in other ways if I go out to the casino. Still go for the fruit machine sometimes, roulette wheel. But otherwise, it's the Internet at home. I like to bet against a kind of system, I suppose, but then maybe that's not true because when you're there, you're focused and you don't think like that. It's the next card, the next roll of the dice, the next . . . , you know?'

'So, your betting is non-sporting, more against, what luck, machines, that kind of thing? Sort of against the system, but not as well.' Clive wasn't sure if he was getting himself ahead of his client. But he was very aware that maybe there was a theme to all of this.

'Pretty much.' Max stopped and reflected on what he had said and Clive's response. 'Something about, I don't know, I don't know what it is, but it sort of feels like it's different.'

'Different?' Clive was unclear what Max was referring to, his questioning tone sought to encourage further exploration.

'There's something about, and this may sound odd, but it's how it feels now I'm thinking about it. It's like I only bet on things that are sort of predictable. And that sounds strange, perhaps, in that I've lost so much.'

'You mean the kind of things that you gamble on you experience as having greater predictability than other forms of gambling?'

'It's like the odds are sort of fixed. You kind of know where you are. How can I put it?'

Clive stayed quiet, he didn't want to disrupt Max's train of thought. It felt important for him to find his own words to describe something that felt important. It felt, to Clive, that this difference was significant as it was in some way defining the limits to the type of gambling that Max engaged in. And it was sufficiently strong to create a boundary; otherwise his client would be gambling or betting on anything. In the midst of something that seemed out of control, perhaps there was something that actually was a form of control.

> Some gamblers do focus specifically on a particular gambling behaviour, others reach a place where they are at risk of engaging in any kind of gambling. Perhaps it is an indicator of the stage of addiction that has been reached? In the case of a problem drinker, they may begin drinking heavily and sticking to a preferred drink, or set of drinks. But in time, as the

addiction becomes more firmly established, the person needs alcohol in whatever form it comes. Perhaps, for the truly addicted gambler, there is a parallel experience, anything that will give them the experience that they crave from the gambling behaviour.

Max continued to think about it. 'I think it's that the chance is more honest, more predictable. You know where you are. You're betting against fixed odds. You know that certain cards will come up, that the dice will land in a certain way, there's a probability and it's fixed. OK, so the odds are no doubt against you, but you're betting on knowing that you *can* win. It's like you have less to think about, in a way. It just feels more straightforward than trying to decide what horse will come first, given the state of the track, the weight, the distance, the health of the horse – so many things.' He shook his head. 'That's never attracted me, somehow. I don't know why. It just hasn't. Cards, machines, that's me.'

'That sounds quite clear, but let me check if I am hearing you right. It feels as though betting against cards, machines, is sort of more honest, predictable, fixed in some way, less other factors to have to think about?'

'It's clearer. It's focused. It's me against, say, the machine, or the dealer. I suppose, yeah, I guess it's more personal and that sounds odd as well, because with machines there is no person, but it's personal to me.'

'It's kind of personal, and the words "one-on-one" come to mind for me hearing you speak.'

'Yes, yes, that's right. It's about me, me winning against someone or something else, beating the dealer, beating the machine, and feeling good about that.'

'The feeling good when you've beaten the dealer, beaten the machine, that's really important?'

Max nodded. 'Yeah.' He had glanced at the clock and noticed time was passing, and it brought him into a different focus. 'I need some ideas to go away with. This is all interesting, and it does feel good to talk like this. Seems like you understand what I'm talking about, but I need to have some ideas, some things to do to change.'

'Mhmm, and that's what feels most pressing just at the moment?'

'It is. I can't have another week of the same. I've got to, I don't know, do something else.'

Clive stayed with what Max had said. Yes, change could often be about doing something else. He conveyed his empathic understanding. 'So the sense you have is that you have got to do something else, something different, this week?'

Max looked out of the window, he was imagining the computer screen so clearly, the cards coming up as they were dealt. He could feel himself focused, the adrenaline, losing track of time and everything as he sat there, seemingly with his bum glued to the seat, his eyes fixed on the screen, his fingers poised above the keyboard waiting for his decision, how much to stake, twist, stick? As he sat there he momentarily lost contact with his sense of being in the counselling room. It was the sound of a motorbike going by outside that brought him back. He looked back at Clive. 'Sorry, miles away again.'

'Pretty intense, when you think about it?' Clive was responding to the sense that he had during the silence of the absorption on Max's face, at least that was his reading of it.

'I was back at home, re-living it. It's so much part of me. Just being at home – I so easily head off to the computer. I can't get rid of it – the thought has crossed my mind – I need it for work. And I need the Internet connection. So that's not an option.'

'So, being at home makes it hard to not turn it on?' Clive did not respond to the comments about the Internet not being an option, maybe he should have done, maybe his response was too directive, and yet the essence of Max's dilemma was his difficulty in not turning it on.

'Even if I went out, I'd have to come back sometime.'

'Mhmm. Still be there, waiting for you?'

Max nodded. 'I need to start somewhere, though, don't I?'

Clive nodded. A phrase he had heard some years back had always stuck with him. He wasn't sure where it came from. He decided to share it as it felt quite present for him, and seemed to have emerged into his thoughts through the connection he was feeling with Max. 'If nothing changes, nothing changes.'

'Yeah, that's true enough. And the longer you put it off, the harder it gets. I have to do something else with my time. I have to get myself involved in something else. I need a woman!'

Clive felt himself smile, he couldn't help himself, the comment had just come from nowhere. Max hadn't said anything about his home circumstances.

'Now there's a strategy!'

'I do, though, I need someone to get me out more. I've got in a rut. Never used to be like this, but it's how it is now. I'm too used to my own company. Funny, that. It all started so socially. But now, somehow now it's different, apart from going to the casino at weekends. I need to address that as well. But I need to get out during the week, get back on the social scene. It's too easy, though, to come home – I often work late at the office – and don't feel like going out. But I'm going to have to do something different.'

Clive nodded, 'mhmm, something about changing your routine in the evening?' The time for the session to end had nearly arrived. 'Seems like that's where we will have to end this week.'

They discussed briefly whether the session had been helpful, and Max said that it had, that it had made him think more and that he'd try and make some changes in the week. They agreed to meet up again the following week and thereafter weekly to try and focus more on making changes as this was what Max wanted.

Clive reflected on the session, on the struggle that Max had before him. What had seemed like harmless fun in childhood had clearly got out of hand, but it wasn't that way for everyone. And yet the increasing availability of gambling must surely increase the risk of people getting not just addicted to the behaviour, but perhaps more importantly to the feelings and psychological experiences that come with it, and the physiological ones as well given the chemicals that could be released in the body during the periods of tension, the winning and the losing.

Points for discussion

- Evaluate Clive's counselling style. How effective was he in communicating the 'core conditions' of empathy, unconditional positive regard and congruence?
- What were the key moments during the session, and why?
- How do you experience yourself responding to what Max has been describing? Do you feel able to empathise with him?
- Does anything surprise you about what Max has said so far?
- What might you take to supervision had you been Clive?
- Write notes for this session.

CHAPTER 2

Counselling session 2: the client tries to change his gambling pattern

Max had tried to make some changes during the week. It hadn't been easy.
He lived in a flat on his own. He'd had a few girlfriends over the years but nothing had really developed longer term. In fact, he found it increasingly difficult
to think about having relationships. He much preferred to be at home, on the
computer. It had been that way for a while now. Even before he'd left his family
home he had preferred to be in his room, or he'd be out to the slot-machines.
That was how it was. In the early days, yes, it had been a social experience,
meeting up with friends, but slowly his friends moved on to other things but
he never really did, somehow. He thought they were missing out, that he was
having the best time. He wasn't so sure any more. It felt like he'd lost part of his
life. Now, at nearly thirty, he had little to show for it. He was getting help with
his debts but they were still mounting.

'So, second session, and I really want to let you take the lead on what to talk
about, Max.'

Max wasn't sure. It had been strange, the last session. It hadn't been anything
like he had expected. He thought there would be lots of questions, and lots of
ideas. But it hadn't been like that at all. In a way he wasn't sure whether it
had helped and yet somehow it felt as though it had, but he couldn't quite
describe how or why. He'd been more open about things than he had before.
And in a way it had helped him to focus on his need to fill his time with other
things. That was what he had taken from the session, that and not feeling
judged, not being told off, made to feel that he had done something wrong.
That had puzzled him as well because he had sort of expected that to happen.
But Clive had listened and had seemed quite accepting of what he was saying,
and he seemed to understand, seemed to be able to relate to him.

'I guess I want to talk about what's been happening since I last saw you. Ummm
. . .' Max paused, trying to decide where to begin.

Clive kept the silence, maintaining eye contact until Max looked away, maintaining his feeling of warm acceptance for Max. The truth was that he did like him,
there was something about him – perhaps it was a sense of vulnerability that
he was picking up on, maybe? He wasn't sure. Or a kind of . . . , no, innocence

wasn't the right word, but it was as though Max hadn't quite taken hold of adulthood, that whilst gambling was serious and generally perceived as an adult experience, somehow the image of Max playing the slot-machines as a child, with his mates, somehow that image seemed quite clear. Something about the way Max described it made it quite real, quite vivid. It wasn't that he had gone into much detail, but it felt so believable in the sense that he could see Max as a little boy in that environment.

'I suppose that I want to sort of tell you more about the past, really, fill in some of the gaps a bit. I sort of feel like I want to tell you more about how things were.'

'Mhmm, how things were in the past.'

Max nodded. 'I mean, I didn't ..., well, in many ways I did have a happy childhood. I had lots of things, toys, you know, and games, particularly play station stuff. I guess I was brought up on it in many ways. And videos. I remember watching videos a lot. My parents seemed, I don't know, they never seemed ...' Max struggled to find the right words. 'They always seemed to care and yet somehow they seemed remote. I had a sister, she's a couple of years younger than me. I think she got more attention. She's married, lives in Scotland with her husband and she's got two children. Don't see her much, sometimes we get together at Christmas, that kind of thing. We get on OK. We talk on the phone sometimes as well. She's been concerned, she knows about the gambling, more than our parents do. She's encouraged me to get help for a while now. Just been hard to accept that I needed help, that something that makes me feel so good is actually a problem. I still don't feel it. I still want that feeling that comes from winning, the buzz, you know?'

'Mhmm, hard to feel it is a problem, still want that buzz.'

'Yeah, but I've tried this week.' Max thought back, 'tried to do something else. After the session last week I went home and was determined not to turn on the computer. Shit, that was a struggle. I really, really wanted to turn it on. I could feel myself giving myself reasons to, and how just because I turned it on it would be for work, I wouldn't have to go on-line or anything. I knew that was crap but eventually I did turn on and I did play a few hands. And I lost, but not too much. And it really depressed me. I felt really bad afterwards, and that was sort of different. I mean, usually it's bad, yeah, but it felt different, felt as though I'd let myself down, somehow, that in a way it had rubbished my coming here, and what was the point in talking about it. Part of me wanted to say, "sod it!", and not come back, to accept that I was a gambler and that was what I wanted to do. And yet I knew that wasn't the answer. That it would get me nowhere. Like I say, I felt quite depressed and had a few beers before falling asleep. That wasn't a good idea either, felt bloody grim the next day. But, well, got my act together, got into work. Busy day, stayed on a bit. Sat there for a while trying to decide what to do. Somehow it was easier sitting at work. You can't use the computers for stuff like gambling, they monitor the sites people access, which is fair enough. Usually it's about porn, but they're also sensitive about gambling sites as well. We've had instructions round about it. Anyway ...' Max lapsed into silence, momentarily losing his train of thought. 'Where was I?'

'Sitting at work, trying to decide what to do ...'

The counsellor has picked up on where Max was in his process and not his final comments which were a diversion by association. Is this directing the client back, or selective empathy, or an appropriate response to the theme of the client as he tries to decide what to do about his on-line gambling habit?

'Oh yes.' Max paused, 'Yes, well, I was thinking that if I went home then I'd be tempted, no doubt about it. But even if I went home late, I'd still be tempted, so it was a case of whatever I did I'd be likely to log on. And I knew that I needed to begin to prove to myself that I could make other choices.'

Clive nodded, 'so, you wanted to prove to yourself that you could choose to not log on, you could choose something else to do.'

'Yes, and so I decided, OK, I'll grab a pizza and go to the cinema. Haven't been for ages, but thought, what the hell, I'll give it a go, see what happens.'

'Mhmm.'

'So I watched a film, it was a thriller, usual sort of thing, nothing special. I tried to really focus on it, but as the film wore on I could feel myself getting more uptight, wondering how soon it would end.'

'Mhmm, wondering how soon it would end.'

'And when it did end, I left, headed home, it was about nine-thirty or so by then, got home about ten. Decided to watch the news. Had a couple of beers, thought it would help me unwind a bit. But I kept thinking about going on-line. I could feel it again, really pulling at me. I mean, really pulling at me.' He shook his head.

Clive responded, 'so having got home later you tried to unwind with a couple of beers but you found yourself being pulled to go on-line.'

'I tried to think about it, what it was that was happening. That's not something I've really done, I mean, not as much as I did then and have done since. And I think that's because of last week, but anyway, so, I tried to think about it. What was it that was pulling me? What was it that I wanted? What would going on-line give me? Was it just going on-line?' Max smiled. 'Well, I knew it wasn't that although that was there, that is part of it. But I needed to just . . .' he shook his head again, 'you know, the feeling was that it was about giving myself a boost after a hard day. There was something about giving myself a reward, doing something that was familiar that I knew I'd enjoy, something for me, but most of all there was a kind of "feel-good" factor to it.'

'So the most dominant feeling or pull was something about rewarding yourself with a "feel-good" experience.'

Max nodded. 'And it was like it was my right, I deserved it, I mean, I really was getting a strong reaction to trying to say no.' Max paused. 'The bugger is that I did go on-line and I won a bit, actually won!' He shook his head. 'In a way whilst that was a good thing, I'm not sure whether it was as it just made me feel more like going on-line again the next night.'

'So you felt that winning made you feel more motivated to go on-line the next night.'

'In a way, that would have been the best time to have lost, so I could maybe have used that to argue with myself, but you know the truth is, and I'm not sure how you'll react to this, but the truth is I know that I really don't want to stop. I like gambling, I like the feeling, I like winning – and you do win as the play goes on, it's just that I seem to lose overall. But it's like, I say to myself – and I've heard myself saying it this week – it's your entertainment. Some people go to football matches and spend a fortune on that, some people spend all their money on clothes, or drugs. Me, I like to gamble. And why shouldn't I? And I hear myself justifying it. And I know that the problem is it's so hard to control.' Max felt so many things, he didn't want to stop, but he did, sort of. And he felt pissed off at having to come and talk to Clive about it, he just wanted to get on with his life, and he knew his life was heading into more financial problems and more chaos if he didn't do something. Yes, somewhere inside himself it all felt pretty desperate, but he preferred to push that feeling away. He didn't feel it when he was gambling, too focused, too concentrated to have time to worry about it. Never thought much about the money, not really. He knew what he was spending, but somehow it felt distant, remote, just numbers on a screen. It was the need to feel himself winning, the relief, the buzz, the exhilaration.

'I hear you loud and clear, Max, you don't want to stop, you don't want to lose what gambling gives you.'

'And that's the root of the problem. If I felt totally and completely knowing that I had to change, and that I wanted to change, then it would be different – perhaps. But I'm not there.'

'The feelings and thoughts you have are not completely dominated with the knowing you need and want to change.'

Max nodded. 'No, they're not. I sort of wish they were, but then I know as well that I don't because part of me doesn't want to change.'

'So you wish you did feel that way but you know that part of you doesn't want to change.'

Max paused. He wanted to express it in a different way. 'It's not that part of me doesn't want to change, it's more that part of me does.' He frowned, thinking about what he was trying to say. Clive noticed the frown and did not respond immediately, respecting the fact that Max looked as though he was still processing something.

In the rush to be empathic the counsellor can cut across a client's process. It is important to be sensitive to what is happening within the client when deciding on the timing of an empathic response, and sometimes it has to be put aside in order to preserve the communicative silence so that the client can remain focused on their own internal process.

Max was still thinking and frowning. What did he mean? The words had come out quite naturally. It was as though, yes, the part of him that wants to change is like a small part within himself which, yes, which primarily doesn't want to change. Yes, it's about which part is dominant. He looked at Clive. 'The way it feels is that I don't want to change, that's me, but within me is a small part that does want to change. But it's small. It's struggling to assert itself because so much of me is fighting against it.'

'Mhmm, that sounds quite clear, that you feel dominated by wanting to continue gambling, yet there is a small part of you now saying, "no" and it is struggling to assert itself.'

'And that's my problem. And I suppose it is asserting itself in some way as I'm here now.'

'So, maybe it has more strength than it sometimes feels.'

'Maybe, maybe. And yet, you know, it's so hard to not gamble on-line, so hard.'

Clive nodded. 'So hard.' He really felt the emotion in Max's voice, of the part of him that wanted to change but was finding it so hard.

'It's like I want to change and I don't. I feel like a war zone. I suppose it won't always be like this, but it feels like it may be.'

'Like it will always be a war zone.'

'Always be a battle with myself.'

'Always a battle between the two parts of yourself.'

Max nodded. He knew he had to change, he knew it was out of control and that he had to rein it back in. In a way he had a bit, he didn't spend as much time on-line as he did. He was trying, whereas before he didn't give it the kind of thought that he did now. But he still did it. And he wanted to do it, and he didn't want to do it, at the same time. 'It really does wear me out, the struggle that is. But when I'm playing, I'm so focused. I sort of get into my gambling self, I guess, and I'm away. I know what I'm doing, I'm in control and it's like, yeah, it feels good, so good. And it is, at the time. It is giving me a good feeling. And going to the casino, well, that adds something else as well, more of a social experience, of feeling part of something, something that I feel quite at home with.' He shook his head.

'You feel quite at home in the casino environment?'

'I do, I really do. It's . . . , no, it's not strange, it's how it is. It feels right to be there, you know, and I said about it feeling like home. It sort of does, feels like it is the place where I can be me.' The last comment Max hadn't planned to say, it came out.

Clive responded to those last few words, 'the place where I can be me'. He used the first person for emphasis, wanting to enable Max to hear what he had said. Somehow, in that moment, it seemed important to do this. He had no rational reason, no theoretical explanation, but the words that Max had used, and the way he had said them, made it feel like they were really important.

Max was looking into space to the right of Clive. He snorted and nodded his head. He felt himself going quiet. "Yes", he thought, "that's it, isn't it? I feel at home at the casino, and I feel at home when I'm gambling, there or at home, on-line. I feel at home". He shook his head, taking a deep breath, held it momentarily and then breathed out heavily. He took another deep breath. 'That's it, isn't it?'

Clive was nodding slightly in response. 'I sense its importance in how you have responded to what you said.'

'Yeah, it is important. I feel too at home with it all. That says it all, it really does. And that goes way back, I think that feeling goes back to those early days with the slot-machines. Still play them, still feels somehow right, yes, there's a feeling of rightness about it.' He shook his head again. 'It feels like I am doing something that feels so natural, so right, so, so . . . , I don't know, just so much a part of me.'

'Mhmm, it feels so right, it's so much a part of you.'

Max took another deep breath. 'This is my problem, such a big part of me is "the gambler", if you like. I have to be something more than that. I mean, yes, I am, I know I am. I'm a software writer, that's what I spend my days doing, and managing. I'm a manager as well. And yet they're not really me. I mean, they are, when I am them. But then it's like deep down, yes, deep down I'm the gambler. That's who I am.' He shook his head again, still staring away from Clive.

'Deep down you are "the gambler".' Clive felt very focused as he listened to Max, though he was also aware that the session was due to end. It felt as though Max was engaging with his own process and sense of self in a profound and meaningful way and Clive did not want to cut across it, but he knew he needed to maintain the time boundary as he needed his own time before his next client.

'I have to be more than that.' Max looked up and caught Clive's eyes. 'I have to be more than that.' Max had also now noticed the time. 'Looks like I must leave with that thought.'

'Seems an important thought to dwell on. And yes, our time is nearly up.'

'I feel somehow calmer in myself. I don't know why because a little while ago I was talking about feeling like I was in a war zone, or did I just think that?'

'You did say that.'

'Hmm. I need to be something more. And it has to be something social, something for my life outside of work.'

'Something social and outside of work, yeah?'

Max nodded thoughtfully. 'I know I talk about not wanting to change, and yes, that's there, and it's big, but I do want to change. The gambler in me gives me a good feeling, but it causes grief, and it gives me problems. I know that. I have to control it. I don't know that I'll get rid of it, it's such a part of me, but I need to be something else, I need to give it a break somehow.'

The session drew to a close and Max left. He was more thoughtful. He had stepped away from his gambling sense of self and was able to look *at* it. He knew it would pull him back into it, it was still too close, too much who he was – he wasn't able to say part of himself for the reasons he'd described during the session. He hadn't any more ideas as to how he would handle his week, but it had felt right to have talked the way that he had. Maybe he needed more time to think? Or maybe he just needed to find his own way. He'd try and have at least one or two evenings free of it. That's what he wanted. But he knew he needed to do something else. He made up his mind to give that more thought, to think about what he could do instead.

Clive, meanwhile, was feeling for Max. He did have a clear sense of the struggle taking place within him; although he knew that he probably didn't have a complete understanding of what it was like. To feel so torn, so much at home doing one thing, and yet knowing as well that you needed to do something else, trying to change the person that you are into something else was one hell of a task. And not something to rush and yet somehow Max would need to maintain some kind of momentum. He felt OK about knowing that Max needed to take his time, and that even though he was still gambling, it couldn't be rushed. He needed to change – stop, cut back – when he felt ready and able, when he was ready to allow some other part of himself to develop and be the focus for other behaviours, interests and activities. And he knew that doing other things would contribute to changes in Max's way of being. The two were linked. He needed to trust Max's process, trust him to make the decisions as to what most satisfied him. The gambling is a major source of satisfaction in his life. But now he is questioning it. That has taken the edge off it. But whether it will leave him seriously seeking something else, and whether that something else will be an expression of change, or a kind of substitute behaviour that remained expressive of his gambling sense of self would only become clear in time.

Supervision session: supervisee learns from his own slot-machine experience

Clive had been discussing some of his other clients with Val, his supervisor. He was interested in spending some time talking about gambling in general as well as about Max in particular. He had already introduced Max, describing his gambling, how it had developed, and how he was struggling with it, and how he was realising his need to be more than "the gambler".
'It really takes over, doesn't it?'
'It's who he is, and it's an addiction. Addicted to being who he is? I know addictions are associated with identity. Gambling for Max is an addiction. I know people debate about what is and what isn't an addiction, but it is, for people that are caught by it they really do become quite absorbed by it, into it. I'm not sure what words to use. And like an addiction, it can and does take over. People spend what they don't have, chasing an experience, again and again.' He shook his head. 'Funny, and I don't know the answer to this, but you know how people who use cocaine or heroin say that they never really get an experience quite like their first use, but they keep trying for it, they keep seeking it. I just wonder whether there isn't something similar with gambling, as if that first win, that first feeling of beating the system, beating the machine, beating the dealer, whatever, whether there is something deep in that experience because it is the first time, and for some people it is somehow so intense that they are, at some level, or through some part of themselves, hooked in some way.'
'Interesting idea, and I don't know, but this is something you sense from clients?'
'Yes, but also my own experience. I mean, I don't gamble, I never really got into that kind of lifestyle, I suppose. Don't know why, just didn't happen I guess. But

it could have done, I think. I sort of feel like I could have developed a gambling habit, but fortunately didn't.'

Val was intrigued, wondering what Clive had experienced, but her role wasn't to satisfy personal curiosity but to help Clive to be fully available to his clients.

'So, the sense of the addictive nature of gambling is partly from clients and partly from your own experience?'

'I mean, as a child, I can remember at home playing cards for pennies, that kind of thing. And I was quite good at it. Maybe they let me win, I don't know, but I think I was quite good. We played pontoon and another game – I can't remember what it was called now, but I seemed good at that as well, but I never felt the urge to take it further.'

'So, you remember winning but not carrying on with it?'

'And I've tried to think back to how I felt. And that's not easy – long time ago!' Clive smiled.

'Yes, I know, you get to an age when everything seems a long time ago . . .'

'Mhmm, well, yes, and I kind of feel that I did get something from it. I remember liking to win, but what I can remember more clearly is hating to lose. You know, somehow, and I haven't thought about it perhaps like this, but perhaps I have a clearer memory of the hating to lose than the loving to win.'

'So, losing was hateful and stands out more clearly than the feelings when you won?'

'I really didn't like it, you know? I really didn't like handing my money over to the banker, or as the banker handing my money out. Yes, I remember it was what we called "pontoon", and I really didn't like losing, I mean really didn't like it. It would upset me, I can remember it now.'

'Mhmm, so, hating to lose, getting really upset if you lost.'

Clive was nodding, and then he thought about Max, 'and maybe that's the bit that I find difficult with gambling, I guess, because for me the natural instinct is probably to not want to gamble because of the fear of losing, yes, I don't want to have to experience losing, so I don't do it. But the gambler rides over that. Max doesn't see losing as a reason to stop. I think he said something about you always go on to the next hand, the next deal, it'll be different. You always hope, you always believe that you are going to win.'

'And you don't feel that, or at least, you didn't as a child?'

'No, but I have to set that aside and listen to Max, to understand how it is for him, and I think I am managing that. I haven't found myself dwelling on my own feelings and experiences in the sessions, in fact, it was the thought of coming here that started me thinking about myself, my own experiences and attitudes, and wondering what I might need to explore.'

'Mhmm, so coming to supervision sort of focused you on yourself.'

Clive nodded, 'and you know, I do see gambling traits in myself, in spite of what I've just said. And maybe it would be helpful to talk about that. I'm not sure where it will take me, but perhaps it may make me clearer in myself in some way, I don't know, but it feels right to explore it.'

'OK, so, something about the gambling traits that you see in yourself.'

'Yes, and, well, it's slot-machines. I listened to Max and, yes, I can remember slot-machines on holidays. Never spent much time there, wasn't the money really from what I can remember. But, anyway, I'll go and play them now. And, well, my partner and I recently started to give ourselves a bag of two pence coins, about a pounds worth each, and we just treat it as a pounds worth of entertainment. We don't really attempt to win in the sense of coming away with more than we started with, but simply buy ourselves a pounds worth of fun, you know?' He shook his head. 'Do I sound crazy?' he suddenly felt as though he was confessing something that maybe he shouldn't be doing, although he also knew that was daft and he could do just what he wanted.

'Doesn't sound crazy to me, sounds rather fun.'

'Well, anyway, we've done this a few times, but we were down at the coast last weekend and we decided to do it again, and I was carrying Max in my head, I know I was. I was wondering, "OK, can I really watch my own process here? What happens for me? What goes on when I start playing? What pulls me in in the first place?" And, yes, I was clear that the idea was to buy some fun. That seemed clear. That felt OK.'

'Mhmm, so you go into the amusement arcade, or whatever they're called these days, to buy some fun.'

'So, we each get our pounds worth of two pences, right?'

'Mhmm.'

'And we start to play on those ones where there's a kind of place that moves back and forward and your coins drop down on it and if you're lucky it pushes coins off the front, I don't know what they're called, but that's the slot-machine we usually go for.'

'Mhmm, I know the ones you mean, and there are different kinds, but the coin goes down, falls flat and gets pushed maybe over a ledge to push other coins.'

'Right, you've got it. So, OK, I'm watching myself. I'm not doing too well. I'm half-way through my coins, and now I'm in a dilemma. Do I move to another machine because I'm losing, or do I stay where I am because I've put so many coins in it I must surely start to get some back because they're building up, looking like they're ready to topple over the edge and give me a payout. And I don't want someone else to come and win "my coins". Yes, "my coins"!' Clive shook his head. 'It's personal, my machine, my coins, and I want them back.'

'Mhmm, so it's become personal, you're wanting *your* coins back from *your* machine.'

'But I'm still losing. In the end I go to another machine, same game, I win a little and I feel good. Yes, I knew it, I knew it was only a matter of time. So I go back to the original machine to try and feed more coins in to get my coins back, but still I don't really win much, maybe a little, but not much.'

'OK, so you're encouraged by the win.'

'But I run out of coins.'

'Mhmm.'

'My partner is still playing on another machine and she hasn't lost as heavily as me, she has coins left and lends me a few, well, gives them to me after I have hung around looking pitiful.'

'Mhmm, she takes pity on you.'

'And I lose those coins as well.'

'So now you have lost some of hers as well as your own.'

'So I can't go back to her, but she's still playing.'

'Mhmm.' Val nodded, intrigued as to what would happen next although she kind of felt she knew.

'So, in spite of my intentions to have a pounds worth of entertainment, what do I do? I go and get another pounds worth of coins.'

'Mhmm, so, you break your own boundary.'

'Yes, or rather, my experience is that I bend it, in fact I expand it to cater for the extra coins. It's OK, I'm in control, it's only a pound. I'm saying this to myself, and I'm carrying a belief that I will get my money back. And I know that I won't. I'm experiencing the split. I'm going to get lucky, but it isn't luck, it's skill. I have to find the right machine and drop my coins in the right way at the right time and I will win. And I also know that I probably won't but that's kept quiet, gagged somewhere.'

'Mhmm.'

'And it's also about my partner still playing. So there is something about other people playing around you as well. I can see how that pulls you back. You stop but other people are still dropping the coins, or playing the fruit machines, and every now and then you hear the tumble of money, reminding you that winning happens and it is just a matter of time before it is your turn.'

'You sound quite passionate about this, Clive, you really did watch yourself, didn't you?'

'Mhmm, I did. And I was amazed at how I could get myself drawn into it, but I haven't finished, it gets worse.'

'Mhmm. OK, so what then?'

'Well, I've walked around these cascade machines, I don't know what to call them. And they seem to me to not have many coins hanging over the edge. So I decide to go for another machine, a betting machine, the one with the five horses and you bet on which colour jockey is going to win.'

'Mhmm.'

'I've got a system. No need to go into what it was, but I believe I have a system that will minimise my losses and leave me with an opportunity to win. Basically, there are two four pence horses (blue and red), one six pence (green), one eight pence (yellow) and one, I think, ten pence (white). I bet on one of the six pence and above horses, avoiding whichever was the last one to win, and one of the two pence horses, the one that has not won the longest. And I get wins, but not enough, I'm still losing, but I am getting wins, and I believe more than if I was only betting on one horse at random. I feel myself being convinced that I have a winning system, and I do, but I'm actually losing. So that taught me something as well.'

'Taught you?'

'That if you win enough, even though you are losing, you will feel compelled to carry on. That actually there is something about the experience of winning that is separate from the money side of it. You're chasing that feeling of winning, of beating the machine. And you keep putting the coins in to try and re-live that experience. OK, it's only a small thing, and yet that compulsion is there. I could feel it. And, of course, it becomes competitive when someone else is playing too. Then you are not only trying to beat the machine, but you want to do better than them as well. You begin to take more risks. You begin to think, "well, maybe if I bet on three horses, keep to the same system and always bet on the highest payout horse". I noted the thought but didn't act on it. But I could sense that a greater recklessness could begin to emerge.'

'So, the greater the competitiveness, the greater the recklessness, is that what you mean?'

'Something like that.'

'OK.'

'Then I start on the fruit machines, two pence a turn, but ten pence at a time. I'm on to the silver. I've lost sight of the one pound limit. I am justifying it because it is only two pence a game, although I am putting in ten pence at a time. I don't win much, but I have now broken through a barrier. I get a bag of ten pence coins. Now, I play a little more on the same machine, but I'm not getting much back, I'm not winning enough. The play is fast, they don't tumble for very long, it's quick to get through ten pence worth. My thoughts go back to the cascade machines, but now it is the ten pence ones. If I win, I'll win more. And I catch myself with that thought.'

'That if you win you'll win more.'

'Yes, and in that moment I am aware that I have split the money I must put in away from the money I hope to take out, in my mind.'

'Mhmm.'

'So, I started out buying fun, then it became a desire to win back my money, then it became a desire to beat the machine, and now I am back chasing the money again having raised the stakes. I am more reckless, two ten pence coins at a time to try and dislodge the temptingly overhanging coins in the machine. I win, but not as much as I have put in. But to stop when you are down with money still in your hand, no, that's not possible. Try another coin, and another. And so it goes on. Until – until a point is reached when something in me says "that's it, stop". And that stop was the part of me from childhood reasserting itself, the part that hates losing, a part that said that I'd basically spent what I would have spent on a meal later in the day. Somehow, that came to mind and that was my brake. But, had I not had that reaction, who knows, maybe I would have carried on, I don't know. But I suppose it was 30 or 40 minutes of play but I learned so much, and realised how easy it is to become caught up in it, how easy it is to justify getting more coins, how big the pull is to get your money back, or to beat the machine and chase that inner sense of satisfaction that comes with winning, and makes you believe you'll win again.'

Val sat with a broad grin on her face. 'You really are passionate about this, Clive, it really did get to you, didn't it?'

'It shocked me, it really did, I learned so much and, well, I wonder whether I could charge it as an expense and make it tax deductible! Research, you know . . .'

'I think you'd be on to a loser there, but it's a nice idea.'

'But it made me aware of just how easy it is, and that was small money, small change, but it has to be something similar for larger amounts. The big jackpot machines that cost more per play and, of course, the other forms of gambling that require higher stakes. I was struck by how I lost sight of what I was gambling, and I can see that that is part of it. Your focus is on winning and beating the machine and you are buying opportunity to have that experience. You are buying something, not gambling, buying an experience, or the hope of an experience. You get the experience, but more importantly, the experience gets you.'

'Mhmm, and it got you.'

'Until that other part of me slammed on the brake. And even then I could feel a dialogue running inside myself. But, no, that hating to lose money cut in and held the day. Otherwise I'd still be there.'

'Still be there?'

'If something doesn't cut in, then I can understand why people continue. It is compulsive and, yes, if you allow the compulsion to control you for long enough I can see how it becomes an addiction. I learned a lot, Val, and I seem to have spent a lot of the session telling you about it. But it really did make an impression on me.'

'I can tell that from the way you have been speaking. You really have talked at length and painted a very clear and graphic picture of your experience. And, so, thinking about Max . . .'

'I suppose it has helped me to get a sense of the allure of it all, the seductive quality. How easy it is to get pulled into it. And then, on-line gambling, it isn't that you're actually handling cash, you're running on a credit card, virtual money that's actually all too real. And then in the casinos, betting with chips, again, takes you away from the money. And I know that for some people they prefer to gamble with real money that, for them, is very much the experience that they seek. But I think that for people who are just beginning to experience gambling, losing sight of the reality of the money being gambled is part of the way you are drawn into it. And, as I say, I think there is a point at which you stop gambling and start buying an experience or the hope of an experience.'

'And on top of all of what you have said are the chemicals released physiologically in the body during the process which themselves generate experiences and can become addictive?'

'Adrenaline rush, you mean?'

'And possibly other chemicals as well, triggering pleasure sensors in the brain.'

'And establishing neural pathways and I suppose the equivalent of salivating when you see the flashing lights or hear the sounds of the tumblers or the money cascading.'

The supervision session moved on to discuss a little more about Clive's expectations for working with Max, the practicalities around the numbers of sessions being offered. Clive confirmed that it was open-ended, that he had no idea how long they would be working together, and that he felt Max would be looking at practical ideas for behaviour change some of the time, and looking at his own process and what gambling gave him emotionally and psychologically.

'He needs space to explore, to really give himself a chance to, well, make of his experiences what he will and, hopefully, seek new satisfying experiences if he decides to cut back or stop the gambling, but he is still caught between knowing he needs to stop but feeling he doesn't want to.'

'And he may stay in that place for a while, and he will need time to explore freely what he feels and what he wants to do, and try a few ideas out if that's what he decides upon.'

'And I won't assume that my experiences are the same as his. That wasn't what I was suggesting earlier. His reasons for gambling are his reasons. There may be similarities, but I will not make the mistake of assuming I understand after 40 minutes in the amusement arcade, but it was just so fascinating and I'm sure it brought me some valuable insight about myself, some of which may have wider application, and some of which may not.'

Points for discussion

- What was therapeutically significant in counselling session 2?
- Evaluate Clive's quality of empathy. How effective was it in enabling Max to self-explore?
- How do you react to what Max is saying about himself, about being "the gambler" and his struggle to want to change?
- What is your own experience of gambling (or not gambling) and how might that impact on working with a problem gambler?
- How did you react to the supervision session? What else do you think could have been taken to supervision?
- Write notes for counselling session 2.

CHAPTER 3

Counselling session 3: the gambling experience today, and in the past

'Good to see you, Max. Come on in.'

'Thanks.' Max followed Clive into the counselling room.

'So, how do you want to use the time today?'

'I've been a bit more successful this week and I've made the decision to go to Gamblers Anonymous. I realise I have to put a brake on my evenings, and, well, that seems like maybe it's a way forward. At least, I want to try it.'

'Mhmm, so go along in the evening?'

'Yes, at least once a week, and maybe a couple of times. I just want to begin to break the pattern. I'm sure I can do it, but I need somewhere to go, be with people, you know? It's not that I feel I'm maybe as bad as some people, but, well, it feels like a place to start.'

'Mhmm, so it's also about being with people.'

'People that I hope will understand my struggle. I think I need that. I feel understood here and, well, my sister sort of understands, at least she tries, but apart from that I don't really talk about it. I don't know, it seems like a good idea and I've talked to them on the phone and, yeah, it felt good.'

'Right, so you've made contact and you feel that's what you need to do, be with people who will understand.'

'But I don't want to just do that. I mean, I don't want to stop gambling but then just spend my time with ex-gamblers, you know?'

'Mhmm, that doesn't appeal.'

'It'll keep me still in touch with gambling. I've thought about this. I can see how tempting that would be, but I'm not sure it's what I want.'

'So, that sounds like you want to move away from gambling as a focus, or anything to do with it?'

'And you know, I mean, last week I know I was really unsure about wanting to change, and that's still there, I can feel that, but I know that it's ridiculous carrying on as I am. And yet, well, and yet I still am carrying on. I can't seem to stop. Whatever time I get home I feel this pull to log on. I can't seem to walk away from it. And I know part of that is because I don't want to. I really know that I don't want to, but I do. And that's me. That's why it's such a fucking struggle.' Max took a deep breath and tightened his lips. He felt sad with himself, about himself, that he couldn't just break free of having to go on-line and having to gamble.

'You really don't want to, but you do, and it's such a fucking struggle at the moment.'

Max was looking down. 'I'm still spending money I should be using to pay off debts. At least they're being organised for me to pay off and, well, some may be dropped, but that just means I can get away with it a bit longer. It's like I know one day I'll have to stop, but it'll be tomorrow, it'll be another day. It's like I, yeah, I really don't want my next bet to be my last ... No, it's not my next bet, it's my current bet, yes, that's what it is. The thought of not seeing those cards being dealt, of not chasing that win, of not getting it and feeling that buzz. It's like every time I do it I don't want it to be the last.'

'Every time you bet you don't want it to be the last time you have that experience?'

'I don't, and yet I sort of have to. Unless I can control it, and I want to believe that I can, and then I think about what people say about addictions, about how you have to stop, and stay stopped. And that feels awful, too much. It's such a part of my life, Clive, to never gamble again, I can't see it, that's the honest truth. And I know but I don't know as well, that I could control it, but I have to stop the daily, I don't know, "fix" I guess.'

Clive listened to Max as he spoke, keeping his focus and attention on his client, observing the distraught look on his face as he struggled to come to terms with the notion of not gambling, of never gambling again, that his current or next gambling experience would have to be his last.

'I mean, maybe I could still gamble a little, but something different, perhaps. Maybe go back to the slot-machines, and keep away from the heavy stakes, just to have a bit of fun, you know? Maybe, maybe I could try that. What do you think? I just can't see how I'm going to stop completely.'

Clive could feel the unconditional positive regard within himself for Max. The intensity of his struggle, his not knowing how to achieve abstinence, unable to imagine it, and now how he seemed to be frantically negotiating for a little bit of gambling, just to keep him in touch with the experience. Yes, he felt for him, and he felt with him.

Max was shaking his head. 'I just can't see it.'

'Hmm just can't see yourself not gambling, just can't see it.'

'No, I can't, I-I just can't. I mean, if I could contain it, just occasionally, maybe, and what I could afford, you know, so it isn't a problem. That's what I'd like, be a kind of, I don't know, "safe gambler", I suppose, not giving myself problems. That's what I'd like, but, well, people don't do that, do they? You have to stop and stay stopped don't you?'

Clive knew that he actually didn't believe in these sweeping generalisations, and that some people could achieve a kind of "controlled gambling" habit, like the controlled drinker, but it varied from person to person and often was linked to the depth and intensity of the addiction or dependence, however you wanted to describe it.

'I think that we have to work towards what is realistic, Max. I suppose that my honest response to what you have just said is that I believe people can control gambling after it has been a problem, but maybe not everyone, and probably other things have to change for that to be possible, but it won't be possible for everyone. I want to support you in whatever you decide to do. I don't know what will work for you, but I want to help you find out.' Clive held steady eye contact with Max as he spoke. He was utterly genuine in what he was saying. He knew it was probably controversial in some quarters, but he honestly believed that if the person changes significantly and sustainably then behaviours can change, and the importance of the behaviours can change as well such that they have less significance for the person seeking satisfaction from their life.

Is there a person-centred theoretical position on addictions and whether abstinence is the only sustainable response? The danger is that abstinence as the only answer would appear to be too much of a generalisation. People get addicted to behaviours because they give them something, give them an experience that has a satisfying edge to it. Whilst the need for that satisfying experience remains, and the addictive behaviour remains the most fulfilling way of achieving it – and often the fastest as addictions can require a certain immediacy in the experience – then the addiction will continue.

Person-centred theory is clear. People move through phases of change that can in general be described as a flow from fixity to fluidity, from being constrained by the effects of experiences and self-beliefs, to greater openness and willingness to flow with experience. An addiction, a habit, is a fixation. It becomes a problem as it begins to dominate an individual's life to the detriment of other areas. So, the presence of the 'necessary and sufficient conditions for constructive personality change' means that the person is likely to shift in themselves in such a way that some of the fixedness is dissolved. The types of fixedness will be linked to the way someone thinks and feels about themselves, and about what they should or ought to do based on the conditions of worth set up in the past and often reinforced in the present. As a client unfixes themselves then what will emerge will be unknown until it happens. This is why person-centred counsellors do not have a specific goal. We might say that the person-centred counsellor aims to offer the 'necessary and sufficient conditions', and the objective in doing this is to achieve 'constructive personality change'. But what 'constructive personality change' will mean in specific terms for an individual will be unique to them and what is important about the person-centred approach and its non-directiveness is the acceptance that what form this change will take in specific terms is unknown. Therefore, it cannot be worked towards specifically.

In terms of addiction, a client may specifically want to work towards abstinence or control, and that is fine, they will hold that direction and the person-centred counsellor will respect that. But, you can be sure that the actual change to the addictive behaviour will be only part of what emerges. There will be other, unplanned changes that will occur, and some areas that will not change – the client will feel satisfied with how they are and there will be no discomfort driving a need for change. But, as a client begins to move towards greater congruent experiencing then nothing can be trusted to be permanent. How far the shift towards greater fluidity will extend is not known. What fixed beliefs and behaviours will start to dissolve will only be revealed as the therapeutic process continues.

'I like to think I can control it. I think in a way I need a break, maybe stop for a while with no set intention to stay stopped, but to try and see what happens and try and get used to it.'

Clive nodded. Yes, he thought, but unless the outer change is underpinned by changes within, it won't be sustainable anyway. That was what he thought, but he knew he had to go with his client, with what he wanted to try and achieve. 'To try and give abstinence a go and see what happens?'

'Gamblers Anonymous tells you that. You have to stop, and I guess, well, I need to get a feel for it, I mean, it's all a big unknown, it really is.'

'And I get a sense from you as you speak of just how unknown it is.'

'Yes, yes, it's like I'm being asked to do something that I just don't do – not gamble. And it's me asking it of myself, isn't it? I mean, you're not asking me to do this. My sister wants me to, I know that and, well, the debt people, they tell me I have to stop. And I can see why, but really it's me. But it's so easy to give myself a reason to continue, just one more deal, you know, just the one, just feel that feeling one more time. It is the feeling. It's not the money. That's part of it, but it is the feeling. And, shit, I learned that when I was really young, you know? And with more and more gambling opportunities out there . . . It has to cause more problems for more people.'

'That how it seems, more gambling opportunities, so more problems?'

'How can it be anything other than that? Take the lottery – once a week, twice a week, scratch cards, it's all gambling. Maybe that's more about winning money, but there are feelings there as well, sitting watching those balls, willing your numbers to come up. I've bought my tickets and still do. Once you start, and particularly if you have set numbers, you can't stop, you daren't. What if your numbers come up the week you don't play them? It's only a pound, after all, and people who have more than one set of numbers, again, they have to continue. And the feeling creeps up on you. I watched myself last Saturday, how I was feeling when the balls rolled. You're there, focused, willing. Nothing. I've won a few pounds here and there over the years, but not as much as I have paid out. But at least some of the money goes to good causes, you know, and some, well, I don't agree with everything it gets spent on, and I don't believe a company should make profit from it. It should be all charitable, non-profit making. But even then it's still encouraging people to gamble.' Max shook his head. 'I'm probably going to have to stop that, but shit, what if my numbers come up after I stop? I'd be gutted, you know?'

'Yeah, gutted, thinking of what might have been.'

'But that's not serious gambling, not really, but it can be. I'm sure some people buy crazy amounts of numbers. But I'd rather stick to something where there are better odds. Maybe I'm a bit more calculated. I don't know. It's not what I think about when the cards are being dealt, you know?'

'Mhmm, tell me about it.' Clive hadn't meant to say that, it had come from somewhere in himself, maybe it was more of a colloquial response, he wasn't sure. Maybe he had unconsciously tuned into a need in Max to tell him about it. Or was it his need to hear? He didn't gamble, what was it that Max had said he played? He couldn't remember. Hmm, maybe his curiosity had spilled out. Max was responding.

'It's just the whole experience. You're sitting there, you're dressed up – that's part of it in the casino – and you know I have thought about dressing up at home as well when I play on-line. And sometimes I have, like trying to re-live the experience at home. Crazy, huh?'

'Feels crazy?'

'Doesn't feel normal, and yet, somehow it does.'

'Part of the ritual, part of what feels right about it.'

'Yeah, yeah it is part of the ritual. But it depends, usually I don't, but on a Sunday evening, then I might. Maybe Saturday night is fresh in my mind and I carry it over. I don't know. Sometimes I go to the casino on Friday nights as well. But sitting there, you place your stake and you're focused, you know the cards you want, they're there, in your head. You believe they'll come up, you're imagining them and imagining how you'll feel.' Max paused. 'That's important, isn't it?'

'The imagining how it will feel?'

'Yes, imagining how it will feel to win. There's the anticipation. You know you'll win, you make yourself believe it. It sort of gives you a sense of winning even when you don't. Yeah, the anticipation, and you're so concentrated. I mean, it's easy to be distracted in life, but there you're focused, same with going on-line. I lose all track of time. I set an alarm now because I'd be at it way into the night. I need something to jolt me back in case I have lost track of time and everything else. It's so concentrating.'

'The way you speak, it sounds really important to you, Max, to have that anticipation.' Clive recognised that Max had been speaking in the second person, but had actually been talking about himself.

'Yes, it is important to me. I get so absorbed, it's so intense, and, yeah, it's a buzz, and it's tiring as well. That's why I have to watch it. I'd be a wreck at work – sometimes I have been. Sometimes I've taken sickies, had to, phoned in and then gone to bed.'

'The concentration, absorption, anticipation, they are all key elements for you.'

'It's like I feel . . .' Max was searching for the right word, but the only words that came to him were those that he now spoke, ' . . . I feel so alive'.

'The gambling experience makes you feel so alive.'

Max nodded. 'It does, it sort of stands out. Work doesn't make me feel very alive, I have to say. OK, I enjoy it, and the money's good, and, yes, it is good to see software coming together and there is a buzz when the product is finished, you know? But, no, it's not the same. Not the same intensity, not so personal.' He stopped to think for a moment about what he had been saying.

Clive had been listening carefully to what Max had been saying and he was wondering what ''alive'' meant for Max.

'So, there is something about feeling alive, that sensation, that's the one you're, what, going back for?'

'I guess so. I need to think about that. I've always thought of it as a buzz, a boost, you know, but thinking of it in terms of feeling alive, well, that makes me think that the rest of my life isn't alive, or is half dead or something, and that feels a bit depressing, you know?'

'The thought that you only feel alive when you're gambling, do you mean?'

Max nodded. 'If that's the only time I feel alive, really alive, then,' he blew out a breath, 'what's that about?'

'What is that about?' Clive knew his empathic response was more than that, his tone of voice also conveyed a definite questioning tone as well. He felt as though he had stepped out of his client's frame of reference.

The question stayed with Max. It actually made him sad. He was quite surprised. 'Makes me feel I've fucked my life up somewhat. But gambling makes me feel good, but there have to be other ways to feel that way, to feel alive, there have to be.'

'Other ways to get that experience of feeling so alive.'

'And you know, I'm back in the past again as you were saying that. The slot-machines, yeah, we felt good, and I suppose felt alive. I mean, it was better than school, and better than going home. Mum and dad, well, they never really spoke much. Don't think they got on. Think they stayed together for us in a way. They split up and divorced a while back now. They were living their own lives, we rarely went out together as a family. In a way, my friends were more my family, apart from my sister, though not then. It was later that we got closer. I think we were both affected. And so, what I was saying before about feeling at home, the arcade sort of did feel at home, like it was our territory. You got used to the sounds, the lights, the smells even. You'd think it would be boring but it wasn't. Yeah, we'd go off and do other stuff, like you do, but we never really felt bored at the arcade. The pain was when you didn't have any money.' Max turned to look out of the window. It seemed to Clive as he sat maintaining his focus on Max that he was staring out into the distance, somewhere, probably back into those teenage years. Was that where it had all started, or was it the atmosphere at home that had driven him to look for some other kinds of feelings, some other experiences, that sense of feeling alive? Was home life and school not giving him that? He sat and waited for Max to speak. It was clear that something was happening for him and he didn't want to disturb the silence that had arisen in the room.

Max was back with the sounds of the slot-machines, even now he could hear them. He liked the ones where you could see the money. But they played the fruit machines as well. You had to get to know them. They were so different. People made the mistake of putting money in without understanding what was going on – when you won, how to nudge, which way the nudges went, what was happening when gamble lights started flashing. You had to get to know each machine.

'It's strange but I can see clearly my favourite fruit machine even now. It made a particular sound. But I also liked those ones you dropped coins in and it pushed money over the edge. But those were about winning money, we spent most of the time on the games machines. Space cadets, grand prix drivers, kung fu fighters, I loved them all. There was that focus again, and, yeah, I really wanted to win. I think I was maybe a bit more serious about it than the others. I'd often be the last to leave, or at least, most reluctant. Even then it was getting to me.'

'So, you'd be the one that hung back.'

'I'd have stayed longer. Nothing much to go home to, I guess. I mean, I had games, and I liked to play computer games, and friends would come over, but I liked the arcade, I liked the, I don't know, like I said before, I felt at home there, I really did.'

'And that was the pull feeling at home, it felt better going to the arcade than actually going home.'

Max nodded. 'Yeah, yeah, that's how it was.' He felt the sadness very present once again, though he had no thoughts to specifically link it to, it was just there, an unsettling and cold feeling inside himself, and a sense of feeling a little tearful.

'Yeah.' Clive paused. The atmosphere had changed, he could feel the shift, he felt his own focus sharpening, as if there was a sudden intensity present, the silence felt somehow almost electric. He knew, from his experience, how this kind of phenomenon could occur and how often it seemed to be associated with a client connecting with something deep and emotional, something significant. He knew he needed to be extremely attentive, present and available. He let the silence continue. Clearly, Max was experiencing something within himself and he had no wish to disturb it. Clive trusted that whatever was happening was timely and necessary. His role was to offer and preserve the core conditions. He felt himself feel a little spaced out; there was a little spacial distortion, Max seemed to suddenly seem smaller and more distant in the room. Clive stayed with the feeling, it had happened before with clients. He stayed still and continued to wait.

Such occasions in therapy are distinctive. They seem to affect the atmosphere. The counsellor needs to be focused, sensitive and open. Often memories are emerging from depth. It can feel as though they affect the fabric of time and space as they emerge. This experience needs further in-depth research.

Max was back in his past, he was heading home, it was a particular occasion although it happened many times, but this one was suddenly very real and present. He was opening the door to the house. His parents were home, and he could hear their raised voices. They were shouting at each other. They often did. But he remembered hearing them making accusations towards each other. He remembered hearing his father saying that he was only there because of Max and Amy (his sister). That she (his mother) needed to get her bloody act together and start being a mother and a wife. His father had then said something that he had never forgotten. 'I only married you because of Max, if you hadn't been fucking pregnant ...' At that point he heard his mother crying and the door opened and she ran upstairs, straight past him. She didn't say a word.

'My father only married my mother because of me, because she was pregnant with me. He didn't love her. I don't know how much he loved me, or she loved me, come to that. I don't know.' Max was speaking without really thinking about what he was saying. His focus was still in the past, and yet it seemed so real, so present, as if it was happening inside him now. He carried on speaking. 'I think I started to hate them both then. I think I sort of decided then that I'd keep away from home. I don't know, I don't know what I was thinking. And I know I was sad, and confused, and didn't know what to do. My Dad's jacket was hanging up, and I went through his pockets and took some money, and then I went back out, back down to the arcade. And I was there a long time, I know that. I didn't rush into spending it, I spent time walking around looking, watching, seeing the expressions on people's faces. Then one of the boys from our group arrived with a friend I didn't know. And we played the machines, and I felt so good, and so awful as well. And I didn't want it to end. I didn't want to have to go home. It was in the summer and it was beginning to get dark. I was thirteen, I think, something like that.'

Clive continued to listen. Max was speaking slowly, still looking out of the window. It was as though he was talking to himself, but talking to him as well. He kept his focus and maintained his feelings of warm acceptance for Max who now felt so much like that thirteen year old boy: confused, sad, hurt, playing the slot-machine with the two boys, and not wanting to go home, wanting to stay in the arcade. He believed in the importance of listening, of attending, that the real empathy was what happened whilst the client was speaking.

There is the empathy that is felt within the counsellor whilst the client is speaking or communicating, and which is concerned with contact, connection, attention and with allowing the words spoken to touch and affect the counsellor's experience. And whilst the counsellor silently listens, there will also be physical communication taking place – facial expression, body language, etc. which the client will receive and hopefully experience as indicating that the counsellor is actively listening. And then there is the communication that follows, when the counsellor communicates what they have heard and understood from what the client has said, and how they have said it. Perhaps it is the listening that is most important, that the client feels listened to as they are speaking, feels cared for when they are feeling and experiencing what is present for them.

'Thirteen, wanting to stay in the arcade, not wanting to go home.'

Max took a deep breath, and closed his eyes. He could feel emotions inside himself that he really didn't want to feel. But he couldn't keep them away. He swallowed. 'I think my mother cared about me, but I wasn't around much from then on, stayed out as much as I could, or when I was home I played computer games, really lost myself in them.'

Clive felt the atmosphere shift again.

'Your mother seemed to care, but you kept away, even when you were there.'

Max nodded. 'Yeah. So, hmm, I guess that was a significant time for me. Something changed. Something was different after that. It was like I'd decided not to be at home unless I had to be, and to have nothing much to do with my parents. Maybe they should have split up sooner. I think maybe it would have been better to have just been with mum. I know it's all a bit uncertain, but I think she'd have been a better mother on her own. And maybe, well, maybe I'd have been different as well.'

'Mhmm, the feeling that if you'd only been with your mother, things would have been, and you could have been, different?'

'Maybe, if it had happened earlier. It was too late by then, I think. I was already drifting away.' Max had turned to look at Clive. 'That came back so clearly, you know, leaves me feeling kind of wobbly inside.'

'Mhmm, powerful feelings, images, thoughts, they can feel like they're happening as you sit there.'

Max appreciated hearing that because that was exactly how it was. 'It's like I could see it, feel it happening just now, even though it was a long time ago, but it was there, with me, still part of me.'

'Still part of you.'

'And it's linked to my gambling, it has to be. Has to be. It's not easy this, is it?'

'No, no it isn't.'

Max nodded, taking another deep breath and letting it out slowly. He stretched his shoulders back a little, it was feeling stiff. 'Oh, I think I've been sitting without moving for too long.'

'You were really lost in thought and feeling, though maybe lost isn't the right word.'

'I was lost, I lost something, and the machines made me feel good. I won that night, I actually won, had money left when I went home. I remember that. Can you believe it?'

'That must have been important for you to remember it so clearly.'

Not a classic empathic response, it is more focused on the sense that the counsellor is picking up on the importance of the experience. The counsellor has not caught the energy of the comment that has been made by the client. A more accurate response might have been, 'Hard to believe, but you won. The machines really made you feel good'. It would have kept the client's focus. What happened was the client was pulled more into the present, into a more reflective place, and away from the re-lived experience.

'Hmm. I learned something that night, didn't I, somewhere else to go, somewhere that could make me feel good, get me away from what I had been feeling. I wonder. I mean, it hadn't been good at home before, but maybe from then on, maybe I was seeing the arcade differently, I don't know, it's a long time ago and I don't remember everything.'

'A long time ago, some things you remember, some things are forgotten.' Clive had glanced at the clock. 'We have only a few minutes left.'

'OK, I'd lost track of the time. Hmm. I feel like I have a lot to think about, Clive, I'm not sure how I'll make out this week. But I think what's happened just now is important. I really feel like I've got things to think about, make sense of, yeah, things to make sense of.'

'Mhmm, things you maybe hadn't thought about for a while, now very much present for you.'

Max nodded, 'yeah'. He paused. 'Same time next week?'

'Sure, same time.'

'OK, thanks. I'm going to cut back again this week. Try to, anyway. I have to find other ways to feel good.'

Max left, still very thoughtful. He hadn't got to go back to work, and he felt he needed some time to himself, but he didn't want to go home. He never felt comfortable at home. Liked to be out or lost on the Internet. He hadn't always gambled when he was surfing, in fact, he would still surf sites now, often to do with work, looking at the way sites were constructed, trying to pick up ideas. And he'd begun to surf for sites that offered support for gamblers, and which had ideas that might help. Now, though, he just wanted to sit somewhere. He felt the urge to head for the coast. It wasn't that far away. It was a little while later when he pulled up on the promenade, and watched the waves rolling in. It was fairly calm, and warm. He decided to go for a walk. Like any resort it had the usual arrangement of restaurants, fish and chip shops, rock stalls, and, yes, amusement arcades. Funny, he felt like he wanted to go in, and yet something was keeping him out. There was still a kind of, he could only think of it as a sort of numbness, that he had felt towards the end of the counselling session, like he was in his own world, just walking along, like in a kind of bubble. Funny feeling. He just kept walking, eventually he sat on a bench and watched people on the beach. He felt as though he had a lot to think about and yet somehow he couldn't really think. He felt sort of muffled, like he wasn't really in touch.

The sensations began to fade. Max had picked up a cup of tea from a stall a little further along. He was further away now from the beach where most of the people were. He sat down again and thought about himself and his life. He had to make some serious changes, or else he'd still be doing what he was doing in ten, fifteen years time. What was that phrase, 'nothing changes, if nothing changes'? He had to move on in some way; had to break free of his gambling. He couldn't avoid using the Internet, part of his job, but the gambling sites he had to keep away from, somehow.

Points for discussion

- How therapeutically helpful were Clive's responses in this session?
- How would you define addiction using the language of person-centred theory?
- What enabled Max to reconnect with his childhood in such a powerful way? How did you react to this, what thoughts and feelings were you left with?
- What would you take to supervision from this session if you were Clive?
- How do you think Max will finish his day? If you were describing the rest of his day, what would it include?
- Write notes for this counselling session.

CHAPTER 4

An update

Max did not attend the next session, he wasn't able to get time off from work. It had become very busy and he talked to Clive on the phone. The sessions were changed to fortnightly.

He attended the next two sessions, and talked about his experience at Gamblers Anonymous. Somehow it did feel right for him to be there, and it was about not having to explain what he felt and what a struggle it was. People did seem to understand. And it did help him to begin to get out in the evening. He made a couple of friends there and they would meet up some evenings, go for a drink, and that felt good. He needed something to feel good about, and it got him out of the house.

He talked to Clive about how he wasn't sure whether he ever really felt good being at home, and wondered whether that also went back to childhood. Or was it being on his own and not having anything to do other than work, or the gambling sites. He discussed his need to have more of a structure to his home life, to somehow start to make his house more of a home, which, he realised, he didn't actually know how to do. He wasn't sure what a home was, other than the place you went to eat and sleep. He began to think about making changes to his home, diverting some money from gambling so he could see a positive result in not gambling it away.

He'd taken the decision to stop gambling. That was in part due to what he heard at Gamblers Anonymous, but it was also something inside himself as well. He could see more clearly how the gambling was a habit rooted in early life experiences. He wanted to give his life some direction, some purpose. He was spending too long looking at computer screens, he knew that. He had to get a life, a broader life. He had to make changes.

He found a really helpful website offering software that blocked you from going on to gambling sites. He'd installed this and it was definitely helping. It was a good page, lots of useful information and tips: don't chase your losses, remember that you are spending real money, keep track of the time and of the money that you spend. But now he was simply not going on-line to gamble. At least, that was his plan.

59

He thought of joining a gym as well, but hadn't done anything about that. Somehow that seemed too much of an effort. He could see the sense in it, but, well, it wasn't something that really appealed. No, he had to control his use of the computer at home, and that meant getting out more. He needed a relationship in his life. He needed a reason to get out, and he needed a reason to make his place more of a home. All these needs, and yet, deep down, the truth was what he really wanted was to carry on gambling. He was changing behaviours, but he wasn't changing in himself, not enough, not in ways that made him really want to do these other things. He was still forcing himself. Not because he was being told to, well, he wasn't being told to by Clive. But he did feel a pressure at Gamblers Anonymous. Yeah, they were keen for him to make changes and he felt he should as he was part of it, and maybe he wasn't being honest with them about how much he still wanted to gamble. He seemed more able to be open to Clive, somehow. He seemed more accepting of the fact that he still wanted to gamble and that, until he'd installed that software, he still had been. In fact, he was still going to the casino. He somehow didn't want to lose that as well, not yet anyway.

Counselling session 7: the gambler within and the not-for-gambling sense of self

Max wasn't feeling too good in himself. The past two weeks hadn't been easy. He'd dropped out of Gamblers Anonymous. He just felt like he needed a break from it. And, yes, he'd uninstalled the software at home. He knew that he needed to talk it through with Clive, at least he felt Clive would understand or at least try and understand why.

'So, I'm back on-line gambling again, the trouble is I'm not enjoying it like I used to, there isn't the same buzz. I feel bad about it, and that's crazy. I like gambling, but I don't. I can't seem to lose myself in it the same now.'

'It's like the experience has changed, no buzz, and you actually feel bad about what you are doing.'

'It's like I know I shouldn't be doing it. I feel like it's something to be ashamed of.'

'Mhmm, ashamed to gamble on-line.'

'It wasn't like that to begin with. I mean, I had mixed feelings, but, no, it felt good, felt like a relief, you know, to have that back in my life again, but somehow that didn't last. And maybe it's because I have been losing more. But then, I'm not as focused as I need to be. I'm making mistakes, I know I am.'

'Making mistakes because you're not focused?'

'Yeah, it's like part of me, that part that we talked about a while back that doesn't want me to gamble, that's sort of more present.'

'OK, so whilst you have begun gambling again, that part is making it uncomfortable.'

'It is. And, well, it's telling me something. I know I have to stop again. I guess this is what happens. But what I want to talk about as well is how I came to start up again. Made me realise how little control I had.'

'Mhmm, is that what you want to talk about now?'

Max nodded. 'It was last weekend. I'd been doing well. Going to meetings and I wasn't using the on-line gambling sites at all. And then, I don't know, it was on the Sunday, I remember getting up and feeling different. It was like I knew I was going to gamble. I'd had a difficult night, hadn't been able to sleep much, and I'd kept dreaming about gambling, and about winning, about those good feelings, you know, the feeling alive, and yet it wasn't making me feel good. I mean, it was, and it wasn't. I don't know. Can't make it out. But when I got up in the morning, quite late because I'd slept badly, I just knew I was going to uninstall the software and gamble. No question about it. And it wasn't as though I really argued with myself, which I thought I would. I've given it so much thought, and questioned what I should and shouldn't do, but this was clear, quite matter of fact in a way. I was going to go on-line and play. It was like I was in another place.'

'Another place?'

> The client has spoken at length but the empathic response simply highlights the last thing he has said. The counsellor is being sensitive to the client's process, not wishing to draw him back. He has conveyed his listening through his attention, he therefore affirms his presence and his attention. The questioning tone is to offer the opportunity to the client to say more, if he chooses.

'In myself. It was as though I was in some other place, I don't know, I was just thinking differently and it was the fact that I didn't feel like I really fought against it. That gets to me now when I think about it.'

'Mhmm, so, you dreamt of winning, had a disturbed night and when you got up you knew you were going on-line and you really didn't try and resist it.'

'No, I just got up and did it. I mean, where was I?'

'Mhmm, where were you, where was the resistance.'

'It wasn't there. And that's scary. I mean, OK, if it had happened and I had felt myself fighting – I, OK, well, maybe I could deal with that, you know, make sure I had some better arguments another time, or try and put up some more boundaries and barriers. But I didn't. I just got up and got into it. And lost, of course.'

'Mhmm.'

'And have been all week, and now I'm here and I need to get that software up and running again to block the sites, and I need to get a grip on myself again. But it's been a crazy week. And, as I say, I haven't enjoyed it. I sit there and I'm not concentrating, I'm not focused, I don't feel the same buzz. I came out of it last night, earlier than I might have done. I guess that was a good sign.'

'Mhmm.'

'Like I'd had enough.'

Clive thought about binge-drinkers he had worked with in the past who could stop seemingly mid-binge, feeling they'd had enough. He wondered whether a similar phenomenon might have happened for Max.

'Did it feel more intense than usual?'

'It did to start with. Couldn't spend enough time on it, but then it began to change, and as I say, by last night, I just felt I'd had enough.'

'Hmm. Sounds like a kind of gambling binge, if that makes any sense?'

Max thought for a moment, 'in a way, I think it does. Maybe it was building up, or something. I don't know. And I'm sure the fact that I had stopped Gamblers Anonymous was part of it, like I was setting myself up in some way.'

'Like you were sort of planning it without being aware you were planning it?'

'Something like that, yes. So I really have to watch myself for changes in the way I'm thinking, I guess. I mean, I really felt I needed a break from the meetings. I seemed to be able to accept my reasons. Felt a bit guilty, but also quite sure as well that it was what I needed to do, that, yes, it was about taking control, doing things my way, proving to myself that I didn't need meetings. That was the kind of stuff in my head.'

'Mhmm, doing it your way and proving something to yourself.'

'I proved I couldn't do it, that my way took me back gambling again.' Max shook his head. 'Does it ever stop?'

'Mhmm, and it takes time. People do lapse, we have to learn from the slips.'

'I guess I thought I was OK, I could do it my way. But I also think that there was something about the gambling part of me, "the gambler", I guess you'd call it, that was sort of fighting back, you know?'

'Mhmm, "the gambler" fights back.'

'Yeah and did he. And now, well, he's quietened down again. It's like he kind of reminded me he was there. It sounds strange talking like this, but it's how it feels, and I remember how we talked about "parts" before and it made so much sense. It's like the gambler in me got hold of the controls and that was it, the part of me that was in control, I suppose got pushed aside.'

'Hmm, so "the gambler" fought back.'

'And it's like he's still around. He's gone quiet, but he's around. I can almost sort of sense him smiling, and it's a very smug smile, a very satisfied smile, you know. Bastard!'

Clive was struck by the forcefulness of Max's voice.

The counsellor has responded to what he sensed to be present within the client's inner world. Empathy is not always about letting the client know what you have heard them say, or what they have described experiencing, sometimes it is concerned with conveying an appreciation of something else, conveyed through the manner of speech, or simply a sense that the counsellor picks up from the client's way of being. It is more likely to be accurate where there is a sense of very definite connection with the client. This does

> not necessarily mean at depth. It can be to something very much on the surface of a client's experience. What is important is that the connection is clear and so what is sensed is less likely to be subject to distortion.

'You don't like him, do you?'

'He's bloody creepy, and he's strong, he took me over so easily.'

'Mhmm, he just calmly took over.'

'Yeah, like he just rode into town and took over – somehow I've got an image from the old westerns you know?'

'Mhmm. The gambler rides into town and takes over the game, kind of thing.'

'That's it. And I know I've talked about it as a part of me, but it is *me*, isn't it? I mean, it's part of who I am; this urge to take over and get into the game. That's me, but it's not all of me. I suppose it's a shock when it happens like this, so suddenly, I guess I'm still trying to get my head around it.'

'Yeah, it can be very disorientating, you need time to make sense of it all and . . .' Clive wasn't sure what he was going to say next. Max finished the sentence for him, 're-group'.

'Re-group?'

'Yeah. It is a battle and I need to re-focus myself, get myself back to the meetings and get myself off the gambling sites. I have to do it, and I have to get back into my routine at home, and going out. It all went pear-shaped this week. I have to fight back.'

'Fight the gambler?'

'Yeah, and I'm back with imagery from the westerns – funny, I've always liked westerns, don't know why. Maybe because there was often a card game in the bar, you know?'

'Maybe.'

'In the western there'd be a shoot out. But, you know, I don't want to kill the gambler, that would be killing part of myself. He's part of me. Yeah, he can be pretty devious, I know that, but he's me, how I had to be. I need him to change.'

'You need to change the gambler?'

'Book him into the rehab, yeah?'

'That how it feels, if you could book him into the rehab . . .'

'Seriously, well, in a way that is serious, but it's like, going to the meetings, you know, talking now, I think I can see what the problem has been. And it's so obvious, but it wasn't. It was the bit of me that wants to stop the gambling that went to those meetings. And it's the gambling part that should have been there. That probably sounds weird, but it feels right.'

'No, it feels right to me, too, hearing you say that. It's like you went into the meeting but left "the gambler" outside?'

'And he's got to be the one who goes in, who talks, who shares. The more I think about this, the more it makes sense, even if it does sound crazy.'

'Mhmm, the gambler has to go into the meeting.'

'And he's got to want to go, and I know he doesn't, but maybe if I keep going, maybe eventually he'll be there too. I mean, he is, he's in me, but somehow I feel that part of me backs away. No, I really do feel that the me that wants to stop went to those meetings, but it needs to be all of me.'

'Mhmm, a real sense that all of you has to be at those meetings.'

'And I know that that part of me is there, I mean, of course it is, I'm in the room and it's part of who I am, so of course it's there, but somehow it isn't as well, it doesn't really engage in the process. And I sort of wonder how many other people are like that, there because part of them feels they should be, or that they need to be, or because someone has told them they must be there, but actually the part of them that should be engaging in the process is sort of, well, in the room, but not, if you see what I mean.'

'You mean like the part that wants to gamble somehow doesn't appear.'

'And I'm not sure how easy it is for it to appear as well. That part of me, I mean, it's been visible here, I think. I've talked of my wanting to gamble, my feeling that I should be able to carry on if I want, and that's coming from the gambler in me. It has to be.' Max paused, something new had broken into his awareness. 'You know, I think that the gambler isn't as strong as he appears. I think he's vulnerable, he has to be. I mean, I started gambling, well, maybe not started, but got into feeling good about winning, playing the arcades at a time when I was feeling vulnerable.' He paused again. 'Not sure what I'm saying here.'

'Mhmm, I'm hearing something about the gambler in you being associated with vulnerability.'

'Yes, in a way gambling gave me strength, gave me a focus, gave me a good feeling, back to that feeling of being alive. But he's vulnerable, that part of me is vulnerable, my vulnerability is linked to its existence. It exists because I was vulnerable. It has its strength because of my vulnerability all those years ago.' Max paused again, collecting his thoughts. 'I'm not sure where this is taking me.'

'Not sure where this notion of the gambler being linked to vulnerability is taking you.'

'I am vulnerable in the sense that I have experienced how the gambler in me can take over, so I am vulnerable to gambling, to the temptation and to the behaviour itself. And yet it formed to help me overcome feeling vulnerable, feeling sad, feeling, well, unwanted – given what I overheard at home.'

'So, the gambler gave and gives you strength, and it sort of takes it away as well?'

'It does threaten to take it away now that I am trying to find a different kind of strength which doesn't rely on gambling to feel good.'

'Mhmm, OK, I can see that. The new source of strength doesn't rely on gambling.'

'So the gambler in me is under threat, and it doesn't like it so it asserts itself and, well, my experience was that the new me, the non-gambling me – or perhaps I should say the controlled gambler me, as that is perhaps more accurate – just didn't have the strength.'

'The controlled gambler didn't have the strength.'

'And, even as I say this, I want to get away from using the word "gambler". Part of the problem is thinking only about myself in terms of, say, "gambler" and "non-gambler". I'm more than those. But it seems like this sort of split seems to dominate. But there's part of me that works, and enjoys what I do, gets a satisfaction from it. There's the part of me that likes driving.'

The client has felt empathised with. The parts of his nature that he has revealed are felt to be accepted and acceptable. This is what the counsellor seeks to convey. However, the client has realised that he is more than the parts of himself connected with the gambling behaviour, and the attempt to change it. He wants to experience himself more holistically and, importantly, wants this acknowledged by others, in particular, his counsellor. He wants to move beyond what he feels to be a gambling-centred focus (simply because that is what he has been talking about) to a more inclusive sense of self. This is also about the client owning a larger sense of self, of his identity, and is a step on the path towards a desire for greater congruence in himself and in his relationship with others and to the outside world.

'So you want to think of yourself more holistically, and not feel stuck with definitions that are simply linked to one area of your life, of your gambling or non-gambling behaviour.'

'There's a gambling me and a not-for-gambling me, I can see that, but I need to be more than my not-for-gambling bit. It's too negative. I can't spend time not doing something. That's my problem. And I've tried to replace it with something else, but I'm still thinking in terms of gambling and not-gambling, and I need to think differently. But I question, as well, whether I am ready for that.'

'Ready to think beyond the gambler/not-for-gambling conflict?'

'And, you know, whilst I know they are in conflict, of course they are, and yet, somehow, both are trying to give me a kind of strength, a way of coping. OK, they take different behaviours, but essentially it's just me trying to cope, trying to find the best way to be. Gambling has been a big part of my life, something I've enjoyed, something that rescued me in a way as a child, gave me a focus, gave me something to feel good about. I needed that. Without it, well, you know, maybe I'd have been into drugs or something else. But I didn't do that. I could have done, it was around, but somehow it wasn't for me. I had something already.' Max felt quite strongly about what he was saying, and as he spoke he felt more convinced by what he was saying.

'So, gambling gave you strength, helped you avoid maybe getting into drugs?'

'I don't know, but maybe. Maybe. But that's not to say that's how it is for everyone, you know?'

'Sure, it's your experience.'

'So, gambling, playing the computerised games and the slot-machines gave me something. But it got out of control over the years, and I can see that. But it still gave me something. And now, well now I'm trying to find that something in some other way, aren't I? But I won't find it by not gambling. Just "not gambling" isn't enough. I have to want to do other things, I mean, *want* to do them, and that's difficult because I guess I've got into quite a rut over the years, really limited myself. And now I have to broaden myself.' He smiled, another thought had come to mind. 'You know, it's something about acknowledging myself as being a gambler who chooses not to gamble, and instead chooses other things.'

Max shook his head. 'No, that's not what I want to say, it's more, "I was a gambler, and now I do different things" ... No, no, I'm playing with words now, getting myself tangled up.'

'Let me say what I think I was hearing before you felt tangled up: that somehow whilst you can acknowledge yourself as a gambler, actually what you want to emphasise now, in your life, are activities that have nothing to do with that.'

'Activities I want to do because I want to do them, not because they are "non-gambling" activities. Yes, yes, that's how I want to express it.'

'New activities that you want to do because they interest you and not because they don't have gambling associations.'

Max sat thoughtfully for a few moments. 'Hmm, and, you know, even in saying that, and I believe that to be right, there's a feeling that, you know, the gambler in me has been a friend for a long while. It'll be a big loss, a big gap to fill. And I don't want to lose that part of me, maybe there are aspects of it that I want to keep.'

Clive nodded. He was fascinated by the exploration. Max clearly had an ease with words and what were in some ways abstract concepts and yet they weren't because he was relating them to his own experience of himself.

'Aspects of the gambler that you want to feel are still part of you?'

'Mhmm. But I haven't thought what, not yet. Maybe that's something for me to think about before the next session.'

Clive wasn't going to in any way suggest Max should focus on it now. He clearly wanted some time to think about this in his own way and outside of the counselling relationship.

'Uh-huh, to try and get a sense of the parts that are themselves part of the gambler.'

'Hmm, yes. Not sure where to take that, but I want to think about that myself. I really want to look at what I can do to bring things back under control in these next two weeks.'

'The gambler' configuration will have a set of thoughts, feelings and behaviours, each might be considered to be a 'part' of the configuration. This may be particularly likely where a configuration within self has developed as such a dominant feature. For instance, 'the gambler' may have different thoughts, feelings and behaviours at the dog track to when he is present in the betting shop. The client may seek to understand how he is in the different contexts. He may not explore them in terms of thinking in configurational terms, this is a theoretical way of understanding a process. The client may speak a different language, simply identifying those aspects of his nature that a particular experience brings to the fore.

One point we must be clear on is that the identifying and naming of a configuration or part is a matter for the client. It is of no help for the therapist to start identifying and giving names to these discrete identities that may, or may not, emerge within the therapeutic process. And the counsellor should not assume that a problem gambler will have a part of himself that he experiences as the gambler either. He may have a different name, he may prefer to associate a feeling with it rather than a behaviour. For instance, it could have been that a client might think of themselves more in terms of a part called 'the winner' and another 'the loser'. Or lots of other possible names may emerge from the client. It is the client's process, and they must be allowed to describe it in their words and meanings.

Clive nodded, accepting Max's wish to shift the focus. 'Sure, what in particular?'

'Well, I'm going to block the gambling sites again, that was working. I'm going back to Gamblers Anonymous. I think I need to. And I need to try and be there in a way that, well, ensures my gambling part is visible. I need to own my feelings towards gambling, that part of me does still want to gamble. I've got to make that more visible. At the meetings I've attended I've either said nothing or only spoken about needing to stop.'

'Mhmm, so, those are two gambling-related actions, and I say that being mindful of what you were saying just now, about new interests free of gambling, or non-gambling associations.' Clive was aware that he was perhaps empathising more with Max's expressed desire to formulate some kind of strategy in the next couple of weeks, rather than specifically to what Max had just said.

'Yes, well, hmm, maybe I'm going to have to go to the gym. I've thought about it, but resisted it. But maybe, I mean, it would be something, wouldn't it?'

'Mhmm, it would be.'

'And a healthy choice as well. Work is a lot of sitting around, and, well, I could lose a bit of weight.'

'So, whilst you've resisted it you can also see some value in going to the gym.'

'Yeah, I think that's what I need to do. After work, before I go home. Maybe I'll be so tired I'll just want to go to sleep!'

'Worth trying.'

'I'll seriously look into that. And I'll think about it as being a straight healthy choice. I don't want to just think of it as a way of avoiding gambling, that's not going to work, is it?'

'From what you've been saying it seems clear to me that you want to make choices for their own sakes, because you see value in them for what they are.' Clive knew he hadn't directly answered the question, maybe he should have, but he really wanted Max to evaluate his ideas for himself. He didn't want to in some way introduce an external locus of evaluation on this important area, yet he also wanted to communicate his supportiveness as well.

'I do. And that's going to be difficult because my life has got into such a rut; work and gambling are the main two activities. Yes, I like driving, and I like reading fiction – thrillers mainly. But that comes secondary to the gambling, or that's how it has been. I listen to music, and, yes, I haven't mentioned this, but I also like game shows on TV. They seem a bit addictive as well, but, you know, trying to do better than the contestants, that gives me a bit of a boost as well. I mean, I'm not a game-show junkie, but I watch a few. I think I could do better than some of the contestants. I seem to have a head for useless facts!'

'Mhmm, so, another interest.'

'But . . . , well, yes, I suppose it is. Hmm. Maybe I should try and get on them. And competitions, I've heard about people who go in for all kinds of competitions, not those ones you phone in or text answers in – they're a rip off, you have to spend so much to enter – the odds will be rubbish and someone is making a lot of money when you start adding up the combined cost of the entries.' He paused. 'Strange, isn't it, me a gambler, but not something like that. But competitions, posting in entries, maybe I could get into that. I keep saying to myself I could do better than the contestants on TV, maybe I should give that a go as well.'

'Seems like you are coming up with a number of ideas, and ideas that have real relevance and interest to you.' Clive felt pleased that Max was thinking things through for himself, and choosing activities that had a certain appeal to him.

'So, I feel more positive after talking to you. I wasn't sure how I was going to move forward when I came in. I knew things had to change, but, well, it's making it happen and somehow keeping "the gambler" in me under control. Funny really. It does feel like I have to find a peace with that part of myself rather than fight it. It's been helpful talking the way we have. I felt quite fearful of how it could take over, but, well, that was what it was kind of created to do in a way. It took over, helped me through difficult times, but then wouldn't move over and let me grow in other ways. That's how it seems now, thinking about it.'

Clive was struck by the clarity of Max's thought. He really did think about things. He knew not all clients functioned like Max, the kind of concepts that Max was handling were not easy, but he seemed to be managing them effectively and making sense of himself, and the choices that he felt he needed to make.

'So, the gambling part of you affected your growth?'

'I think it became more and more of my life outside of work. And before I started work, well, it really did take up my time, either playing the machines for money, or for entertainment although, as I said, it was I think more about chasing that feeling of being alive that came from winning, or the thought of winning, of beating the machine, the game, and anyone else whose scores were listed as being highest. I always wanted to get my name on the top and I'd really work at it. Really work at it.'

'Mhmm, having your name on top.'

'And I achieved it, not all of the time, but my name was up there and, yes, I did manage to hold the highest score for some games, for a while at least.' Max paused as a thought struck him. 'Guess I'm a bit like that at work as well, with the software design. It's got to be the best, and I do put extra time into it, and I push people. Hmm, guess there's a link there.'

'You have a sense that the same drive to be the best also gets expressed in your software design?'

'I'm sure of it. Hmm. Well, that's a good thing, I guess, so long as I don't stress myself out over it. Which I don't think I do. Or maybe I do and the gambling, I was going to say, helps me relax, but it isn't relaxing really, it's so intense, but, well, maybe it's that feeling at home with it that is then so important.

It's something I feel at home with, at least, I had been. This week's been different. I really think I am beginning to change, slowly, but I have to work at it.' He looked at the clock. 'My time's up. Need to head off. Thanks, Clive, it's been really helpful. And I'll think about "the gambler", and think in more depth about who he is and what he gives me.' He nodded to himself thoughtfully as he finished his sentence.

Counselling session 8: gambling satisfaction – more than just winning

Max had begun the next session describing his week. He'd joined the gym. In a way that had felt quite a big step. It was something new. He'd rationalised the cost against what he was gambling and losing. He'd also blocked his access to gambling sites and was keeping himself away from the casino. So he'd had pretty much a clear couple of weeks, except for a few scratchcards, and he had played the lottery. But he did both with more awareness of what was happening. He was pleased with that.

'It was like I could watch myself, like I was giving myself permission but I had control over it. There was a temptation to buy more once I knew I hadn't won with the scratchcards, but I had made myself leave the shop before I scratched them. I think that helped. And that wasn't easy. They sort of wanted me to play them straightaway.' He shook his head. 'What am I saying? *They* wanted me to play them?' He shook his head again. 'And yet, that's what it felt like, like they were kind of calling me, nagging at me. I know it was me, in my head, "the gambler", I guess, desperate to get his hands on them, but I sort of made it clear to myself that I would play them, but not until I got home. It felt as though I was in a way compromising, no, I mean negotiating, with myself. But I think it helped, somehow. I think it's like I need to feed "the gambler" but not too much, keep him happy. If he knows that I'll have an opportunity to chase that feeling, then he's quieter although there still is that nagging pull. It's about the immediacy, and maybe that's what comes with my style of gambling. It's all immediate gratification, isn't it? Not like betting on horses, setting up an accumulator and then having to wait. You stake your money, the cards are dealt, and it's there, happening, straight away. The same with the slot-machine. And the scratchcards as well. Anticipation and then gratification in rapid succession.'

Clive was listening carefully to what Max was saying. There was so much insight. 'Seems like you are forming a relationship with "the gambler", if I can put it that way, and learning to manage that urge for immediate gratification.'

'I've been thinking about that and, yes, it's true. My style of gambling is immediate, a short period of anticipation and, well, then on to the next bet, the next stake, whatever I'm doing. And when I gamble as well I know that the amount does impact sometimes on the intensity of the experience. Not always, but often. The more that is riding on something – and usually it's because I have a sense of a better chance of winning, whether it's the cards I've been dealt, or just whether I feel lucky, that has a part to play as well. If I feel lucky I'm probably more reckless. And if I'm desperate because I'm losing, the same happens. Yes, that's strange, but it isn't. The more intense it is, the more that's riding on it – money, level of anticipation – then maybe I am more reckless. That's why it can be good to have a system, but they're not always easy to stick to.'

'Sure, it's like the system puts a boundary on your gambling behaviour.'

The counsellor conveys a general understanding of what the client has said – simple and focused, and the client is enabled to immediately acknowledge whether he has captured the essence of what he is saying, or not. Long and rambling empathic responses can simply leave the client confused. If the counsellor keeps it simple and focused then it is easier for the client to know whether they have been heard and understood, and can agree, move on, or repeat what they have said. But they are not left sitting listening to a lengthy monologue from the counsellor that will cut across their flow and be likely to leave them out of touch with the point that they had reached.

'And sometimes it does, and sometimes you justify to yourself a reason for breaking out of it. But if you do that then you have to force yourself back into it or you can lose your focus again.'

'Mhmm.' Clive nodded and was aware of thinking to himself how disciplined the gambler had to be, and it reminded him in a strange way about how he, as a person-centred therapist, had to be disciplined as well. He had a system that he worked to. An idea came to his mind. Now, there was a thought for later. He put the thought aside but sought to make a mental note to pick it up again after the session.

Max felt that for a moment Clive had lost his focus, and then it was back again. In the casino there were times when you needed to study the faces of others around you, and he had played poker in the past and he could observe people quite closely when he needed to. 'Like you just did.'

Clive smiled, 'yes, a thought had struck me about how in a way maybe it's a gamble me offering you therapy because I don't know what the outcome will be.'

The counsellor is transparent in his response. He knows he drifted into his own thoughts, and he voices them. Counsellors do drift, it happens. What is significant is the way that it is handled. In this instance, the client is perfectly right. Yes, the counsellor has to verbally put their hand up and say yes, you're right, that's what I did. As to how much explanation is given as to the reason is then a matter of professional judgement. Was the something that took the counsellor's attention likely to be relevant to the session? Should it be voiced whether it is relevant or not? Say it's something that you suddenly remember you forgot to get during the lunch-break, and need to get after work. Do you say what it is? Do you say you thought of something to put on your shopping list? The counsellor may seek to avoid being honest, saying that it will affect the client, disrupt the therapeutic focus. Maybe, but it will inject a certain note of realism into the session as well. And the client may experience a strong reaction, and may verbalise it. So be it. That has to be heard and warmly accepted as well. And yet, this is not a case for verbalising anything and everything that comes to mind. In this instance it is relevant, the client has noticed the counsellor lose his focus. Out of respect for the client, and for the relational process that is at the heart of person-centred practice, an open and honest response is required.

'I thought it was a bit more scientific?'

'Well, yes it is, in a way, but I don't know from client to client how helpful it will be.'

'Hmm, well, it feels helpful to me. I'm pretty much off the gambling at the moment, and I've gained a better understanding of myself. And I know I'm not out of the woods yet. I've learned that from the meetings [Gamblers Anonymous] that you can't let down your guard. They described what I experienced as simply my being too confident, and that I left myself open to allow my addiction to re-assert itself. I didn't talk to them about what we've been talking about. Somehow I wanted to keep the idea of "the gambler" to myself, but I did manage to actually make that part of me more present, sharing with them how I still felt the urge to gamble and what it gave me. That felt important, owning that, and seeing a lot of nods around the room when I was speaking. I don't think I'm alone in this by any stretch of the imagination, but I'm not sure that everyone thinks of it quite the way that we do, here.'

Clive was struck by the sense of a kind of split and yet how Max was trying to work his process in the two settings. He felt he wanted to check out how that was. He knew that clients could find this kind of situation confusing, particularly if they were picking up on different ideas which were contradictory: 'I'm left wondering how that is for you. Almost using one language here and a different language there.'

Max nodded. 'Good point, but it seems OK. Feels more psychological here, more about behaviour there. That's a bit of a simplification, it isn't quite that simple, there is overlap, but I feel I can manage the difference. It's good to be with people who have been there, and some probably are still there, you know? You don't feel so on your own with it, and there are people you can call, talk it through if you feel really tempted. I didn't do that three weeks back, I'd already decided to break the connection and do my own thing. And I can see that was part of the build up to my relapse.'

'Mhmm, so, you find both helpful. That's great.' Clive was genuine in what he felt. He believed people needed support in different ways, particularly when dealing with a deep-seated addictive behaviour. What was important was that whatever they chose to do felt right or had meaning for them in some way. Doing things for the sake of it he wasn't convinced long-term was always the answer, unless someone then developed a genuine interest. But, as had been explored in the earlier session, there was a need for something other than simply trying to 'not-gamble'. Although Clive was also aware that for people at a very early stage of changing an addictive behaviour, that was all they could try and manage simply because nothing else did really give them much interest, particularly if there were depressive symptoms present as well – which could also arise out of the loss of an addictive behaviour.

'So, I'm making changes and trying to stick to them. And, like I say, I've owned up at the meetings about my still wanting to gamble. Funny, that had seemed quite a hard thing to say but it was so well received. It was like I said something that everyone already knew, yet I'd been fooling myself into thinking it was something I shouldn't admit to. You meet people who have been gambling-free for five, ten years – even longer – and you think that they're way beyond feeling an urge to gamble, but people have said that it can still be there, they still have to monitor themselves a bit, keep in touch through the meetings. I sort of thought it went away.'

Clive held back from a smile because he knew what he was smiling about, and he knew it was a personal view although he had heard others talk of the same thing in relation to twelve-step programmes such as Gamblers Anonymous and Alcoholics Anonymous. He felt people could get stuck in the Prochaska and DiClemente 'cycle of change' maintenance phase (Prochaska and DiClemente, 1982). The sense of 'once an alcoholic, always an alcoholic' came to the fore, and addictions were sensed as incurable diseases. Clive didn't go with that. He saw people who could and did change, and he would always argue passionately that it was about the degree of personality change that took place through therapy, or through life experience. He quite accepted that people didn't only change in constructive ways through therapy.

> Much of this debate hinges around the notion of 'recovery'. Is the gambler who has stopped gambling perpetually 'in recovery', or can they reach a point at which it can be said that they have 'recovered' and have freed themselves from that particular addictive tendency?

'You felt that you would, at some point, stop feeling the urge to gamble?'

Max tightened his lips and frowned, breathing and as he was about to speak, just let the air out. He took another breath, shaking his head as he did so, 'I don't know. I don't know that I thought I'd necessarily lose the urge to gamble. It's about control, and whether I'll always feel the urge to gamble in a way that I lose control, that I guess, well, whether that's a problem. That's what I question. Maybe I'll always like the idea of a gamble on something, and maybe I can control that, and maybe sometimes I will, and sometimes I won't, but I'll be in control. That's what I want, to be in control and not feel something in me, well, "the gambler" is taking over. Hmm, so I guess we come back to "the gambler" again. Whilst that's still part of me, maybe I'm still at risk, and yet I can't see myself never feeling like gambling, and so, well, for me to feel that then "the gambler" has to still be there, which means I'm still at risk of relapsing. Something like that, anyway.' For Max the thought that he'd never feel like gambling just seemed too far-fetched, but then, not everyone who gambled occasionally had a gambler inside them like he did. So . . . He wasn't sure. He was still thinking about it when Clive responded.

'It's like will you always be at risk simply because you might sometimes feel like gambling, however controlled that might feel? I'm not sure if I'm getting it right.'

'I mean, people gamble, and not everyone has problems with it. People can take it or leave it, buy their weekly lottery ticket and not be tempted to buy more, perhaps they might bet on the Grand National, but not on any other horse race, or drop in the amusement arcade now and then and entertain themselves, probably lose their change but it's not a problem, they walk out, have an ice-cream and forget about it, you know?'

Clive nodded. 'Yes, people can take it or leave it, it doesn't dominate them or their lives.'

'No, it's not that important, bit of fun, and that's as far as it goes. Now, to me, and I can feel myself reacting to what I've just said, to me there's something pointless about that.'

'Pointless?'

'It's like, what's the point? I can't relate so much to the Grand National, not my thing, but it would be like someone going into a casino and, say, playing a couple of hands of black jack. You wouldn't do it. It's not how it works. It would be like, well . . .', Max thought about it. 'Yes, I guess it would be like an alcoholic drinking a can of beer and saying "great, that's all I need, now I'll go and do something else". It's not like that. You have one but you'll want more. I have a bet and then I want another. More than want, you know, in that moment I *need* another. One bet is not enough, even if I was to win, that wouldn't be enough.' Max was struck by what he had said. It was something he knew, but saying it somehow it suddenly made an impact on him, like he was seeing it differently for the first time. He felt goosebumps on his back and neck.

Clive had watched Max's facial expression change. He looked as though something new had come to mind, though quite why he thought that he wasn't exactly sure.

'Something struck you?'

Max nodded, 'yes, yes, it's so clear, so obvious. Yes, it isn't about winning, I mean it is, but it isn't. If it was then I could stop, or if I won the first hand. But no, it's about reaching some . . . , I don't know, threshold of winning, some kind of level. I don't know quite what I mean.'

Clive nodded and responded, hoping his empathic understanding might help. 'Some kind of level of winning?'

'Yes, but it isn't about the amount, I mean in a way it is, but it's about satisfying something inside me, yes, and until that's satisfied I'll keep gambling.'

'OK, OK, that sounds clear, it's about satisfying something inside you, and that involves some kind of *level* of experience.'

'It's like, yes, it's like it builds up in some way, yes, and each time I'm looking for it.'

Clive was struck by Max's switch into the first person. He didn't often talk in the first person. In fact, thinking about it, he rarely did. So this seemed significant, a significant shift, a significant ownership of the experience. Now it wasn't some generalisation, it was his, what happened for him.

'So you're looking for some particular level of satisfaction?'

'But not consciously, I'm not deliberately setting out to and yet in a way I suppose I am, I must be, but I'm not aware of it, am I? I just do it.'

'So, you just do it.'

'And that's why there's no control.'

'Because until you hit that satisfaction . . .'

'. . . you have to keep going. And it's hard to hit.' Max smiled. 'Maybe you can't hit it, or when you do, well, you have to hit it again, another night, or the same night.'

'Mhmm, you have to hit it.'

'Yes, or else, well, going back to what I was saying earlier, what's the point? The idea of one bet, one deal, it's not enough. Even a big win, it's not just the money, it's about feeling you've won, and you need more of that feeling. Money adds to it, yes, the amount adds to it, but it's not just that. It's like it builds up, you know?'

Clive was aware of drinkers, binge-drinkers, needing to get a certain amount of alcohol into their bodies in order to reach some threshold of being alcohol-affected, whether it was to numb a pain or release an anger, or simply to black out. Yes, he'd heard problem drinkers say they wouldn't bother if there were only a couple of cans, there'd be no point, although they'd probably drink them anyway, but they'd know it wouldn't satisfy them. Maybe something similar happened with gambling, even though it wasn't a chemical fix in the same way except that, of course, it was because the feelings of being alive and of satisfaction are linked to the chemicals released in the body hitting the pleasure receptors in the brain.

'Mhmm, build up of something in the system, inside you.'

'And you have to keep going to hit that satisfaction level. Makes me think of the Rolling Stones, "Can't get no . . . satisfaction." But that's it. Can't get enough to get that satisfaction. That's how it is for me. "The gambler" needs a certain amount, if you like, to settle down. I need it, but I don't, I just feel like I do, and it keeps me gambling.'

'Keeps you gambling.'

'Or it did. And now, well, now I need to accept that I'm not going to get satisfaction like that, I need other ways. And it's back to that feeling alive. That's what did it. I felt good, felt alive all those years ago. Something I was good at, something I could win at, something that really focused me, excited me, all that stuff. And even talking about it now, well, you can probably tell from how I'm speaking, it's still alive to me. That's why it's such a bugger to shift. And I don't want to. I want to feel alive, feel good.'

'You want to feel alive and gambling got you there.'

'Hmm, sometimes. Of course, often it didn't but you go back to it because it has done, and still does sometimes, you're chasing it, all the fucking time man, you're chasing it.' Max took a deep breath and gritted his teeth. 'I've got to refocus this urge. OK, I like to win, I like to beat machines, I need to do that in the gym, don't I?'

'Push yourself, reach goals, you mean?'

'Yeah, but it's more effort, more physical, not like trying to get a higher score on a computer game or getting the right cards and making the right bet. That's not physical. Yeah, you concentrate, but it's not a physical effort. That'll be my problem, making myself make the effort.'

'The physical side of exercise doesn't appeal?'

'If I'm honest, no, but then, well, I've got to make other choices.' He took a deep breath. Max was thinking again about 'the gambler' inside himself. 'You know, "the gambler" just wants to feel good, it's just that he, I, learned a way of getting there that's now giving me problems and, if I'm honest, has done for a while. He/I have to learn other ways.'

Clive nodded. 'Seems to me like in the last few minutes you have really touched something important, and somehow it feels to me that you are really owning it.' Clive was thinking as well about Max's continued use of 'I' in what he was saying.

'It feels personal, somehow, I mean differently personal. You know, and this'll sound strange, but I suddenly feel like I've kind of woken up, in a funny kind of way, I feel a bit more alive, like I've, I don't know, cleared away some fog in my head. I don't know how it happened, or when it happened other than it was about this sense of having to hit some kind of level of satisfaction, like hitting a button, you know, like those, what were they called, at funfairs, you wallop something with a mallet and it shoots a ball or something up a pole which hits a bell if you've hit it hard enough. Except that it isn't all on one hit, each hit builds it up, or you have to hit it enough times, once isn't enough, or something. Maybe that's not such a good analogy.'

'So, OK, the mallet and the bell don't feel too helpful, but you feel clearer now, something has shifted.'

Max took a deep breath. 'Yes. Yes, somehow something feels different. I just know I feel different even though it's hard to explain.'

'You know you feel different but to put that difference into words . . .'

Max shrugged. 'Something's happened. I can't explain it. It's like freeing myself up, or being freed up in some way.'

'Mhmm, feeling freed up, freed from . . .'

'From being in a fog with it all. I need to feel good, yes, fine, of course, I knew that, but it's like now I really know it. And I need new ways of getting that feeling. I fooled myself, gambling didn't really give me that feeling, not really, not often, anyway, but because it had in the past I kept at it. And then, yes, the behaviour becomes part of your life, it became part of my life. It was what I did. And maybe still could, who knows? Maybe it's still there, but at the moment it feels like it isn't. I guess the behaviour becomes a habit and, well, we all get stuck in habits, in ruts. Mine was gambling. And that isn't to say I'm out of it, or if I scramble out won't fall in again, but I have to avoid the ruts. I need to take another path, maybe, one that . . . , no, no, gambling's out there, all around us, I've got to learn to choose to do other things, and learn to want to do other things.'

'You really have shifted, Max, I can see it, hear it, and yes, you're right, the ruts are still out there; maybe "the gambler" remains and still has to be kept an eye on.'

'I think he needs to learn other ways to feel good. He helped me feel good when I felt shit. I should be grateful, and I guess I am. I sort of need him, but I need him to be different. I need me to be different. And it's like maybe I'm now beginning to see it, more clearly, more immediately, more personally.'

'I'm really struck by how energising this dialogue feels. I can feel something's very different. So, what you're saying is that you are seeing your need to be different more clearly, more personally, more, what was it you said?'

'More immediately.'

'Yes, more immediately – sort of maybe more in your face?'

'More in my head, more like!' Max paused. 'Is this what happens in counselling?'

'It can do. Sudden bursts of insight, then, well, then it has to be lived.'

'Hmm, yes, like being shown what to do but then you have to go out there and do it?'

'Something like that.'

The session drew to a close. Max never spent time exploring his thoughts about 'the gambler' that he'd had since the last session. But that somehow seemed unimportant, at least given how he was now feeling. Maybe that would be something he would come back to.

* * *

Clive sat for a moment after the session; it had been intense and incredibly energising. He remembered the thought he'd had earlier in the session. It suddenly seemed a long time back now. But he did want to pursue it. The gambler has a system, it's his discipline. So did he as a counsellor. His system was person-centred theory and the requirement of 'the necessary and sufficient conditions' to provide a basis for 'constructive personality change'. So, he thought to himself, let's run the analogy a little further and see what happens. The gambler gambles to get a good feeling, the anticipation, the excitement and the experience of winning, and there can be other pay-offs as well; for instance, the social experience. OK, he thought to himself, that seems pretty clear. The outcome is uncertain, but winning is possible, it can happen.

He thought of the concentration that could be involved, thinking particularly about black jack on the Internet, or any other card game – poker, for instance. People followed systems, they were focused, concentrated, trying to get into the minds of those they were playing against. Hmm. Intense stuff. Disciplined. He kept coming back to that word. Also, that there was no certainty of outcome, but everything was geared up to the possibility of a win.

So, Clive turned his thoughts to therapy, and to the person-centred approach. Was he gambling with his clients? This was the thought that had struck him during the session. Yes, he had a system. Yes, he had a purpose in what he was doing. He was concentrated, focused, and might sometimes step out of the system, maybe by choice, sometimes it happened, and that would end up as a supervision issue if he noticed it. But he was basically coming into the therapeutic relationship with a belief, that when a client experiences the presence of the core conditions, then they are likely to move from incongruence to congruence, and towards more satisfying choices for themselves, or to a clearer appreciation of the background to the choices they are currently making. He believed that by offering certain therapeutic conditions then constructive personality change would occur, although the exact form it would take would be a matter for the process itself. So, was this a gamble?

It was informed. He felt it was scientific. Research showed people experienced constructive change as a result of person-centred counselling, and other forms of counselling as well, of course. Yet it wasn't predictable, not really. You didn't know when you started a new therapeutic relationship what would happen. But was there a sense of 'winning' if the result of offering therapy led to constructive personality change in the client? Yes, probably. And yet he felt a reaction against the notion that therapy was a kind of gamble. And who was the gambler? He hadn't thought of that. He'd been thinking of the counsellor, that he gambled with what he offered in terms of a non-directive, relational therapeutic approach as being something that would have a beneficial effect on or for the client. But was it the client who was gambling, gambling with their psychological state? He thought of a dice being thrown. If say the higher the number thrown, the greater the constructive personality change achieved, what was his role? To load the dice? He could see that. He could see that worked as an analogy. The core conditions provide the loading, so long as they are communicated and received.

There's a paper in this, he thought to himself, though he wasn't sure quite where to start. Another thought struck him. If therapy is a gamble, and the client is gambling with their psychological state, there could be an addiction to therapy issue to consider, the client desperately seeking to play the therapy game simply for the experience. And if they know they are doing this then they are in some sense congruent to their experience, and if they attend therapy without incongruence then one of the conditions is not present. The counsellor keeps dealing/empathising and the client keeps playing/talking. It would be up to the professionalism of the counsellor, perhaps, to acknowledge what was happening. And at what point would it become unethical to continue, would it be an exploitation of the client's addictive need? Is it unethical for a person-centred counsellor to offer therapy where the client does not have an apparent incongruence? Except that there is always some degree of incongruence, however small it might be, so there's maybe always scope for something constructive and helpful to emerge from a person-centred therapeutic relationship.

Clive decided to cut short his train of thought. He could feel himself being pulled into a minefield on this one, and yet there was something about the whole metaphor that felt like it had meaning. And, with a client with a configurational state called 'the gambler', what did that mean for the client 'gambling' with therapy, or the counsellor 'gambling' with his theoretical system? Or was this simply inappropriate language to use?

Points for discussion

- Evaluate Clive's empathic responding in sessions 7 and 8.
- Where do you feel Clive may have been unhelpful in his responding, and why? Where might different responses have been more helpful, therapeutic, or more in line with person-centred theory?
- Did Max's description of 'the gambler' match any image that you had been building yourself?
- How do you view the notion that gambling is more than just about winning for some people? What other psychological feature(s) of gambling can you identify that might make it attractive to a person?
- What were the key moments during these two sessions, and why?
- If a feature of 'constructive personality change' is movement from fixity to fluidity, can you see evidence of this happening in Max? Is he becoming more congruent? Give examples.
- How were you affected by Max's insight regarding his need for a threshold of satisfaction to his need to feel good, feel alive?
- 'Therapy is a form of gambling' – what are your thoughts, feelings and reactions to this reflection by Clive?
- Write notes for these sessions.

CHAPTER 5

Progress so far . . .

Over the next couple of months Max continued with his counselling. The eighth session had proved to be something of a turning point for him, although that hadn't meant that it was plain sailing. The pull to gamble was still there, that urge to go back to his habitual method for getting that sense of satisfaction. He had avoided gambling on the Internet, and was pleased with that, but he had allowed himself to slide into a pattern of playing computer games, though not to the degree that he had previously been logging on to the gambling sites. In his own mind he felt he could justify this, it wasn't affecting him financially and he was getting a good experience from it. He'd discussed it with Clive, and as a result of exploring it further Max had realised that whilst it was reducing the harm, it could become habit forming. He had noticed how there were times when he wanted to get back home from the gym to log on. He knew that wasn't a good sign. He didn't want to let his life become dominated once more by the computer screen. He wanted to get away from that. Yes, the gym was helping, it was giving him a focus, goals to achieve, but somehow it wasn't the same.

He wasn't going to the casino any more. That had not been easy. He felt caught between wanting to keep that going for the social experience yet knowing that it really was keeping him in touch with that gambling urge, or at least, with gambling as a method for getting what he wanted to experience inside himself.

He had wondered about changing his job. The software that he worked on was for businesses wanting to monitor their productivity and for organising their distribution of goods, that kind of thing. He wondered whether he should maybe think about working somewhere where he could write for games. That felt as though it would bring him a lot of satisfaction, and he was also aware that it could easily take over his life. He'd been there with the gambling. He didn't want to end up with something similar, albeit something he wasn't going to get into debt over.

So, he had reached the decision that he simply had to extend his life and his interests, get out more. The gym helped but wasn't enough. He had got into competitions and had actually won a couple of prizes, so that was encouraging. But that was something he did in isolation. He needed to extend himself and as he sat in the waiting area he was thinking about that session a couple of months back when he had really felt he'd made a break through, when he had felt able to see things so clearly. It had faded since then, it was hard to maintain the momentum, yet he knew that he had changed but he needed to persevere. It wasn't easy. It was hard enough making changes, and he had managed that, but maintaining them without slipping back, that was an on-going grind. He was glad that he had the counselling and the meetings to go to. He felt sure that had he been on his own with his feelings he'd have slipped back. Well, he probably wouldn't have made many changes in the first place.

So, how could he recapture the drive that he had a couple of months back? He thought back. All about finding ways of satisfying that need to feel good, feel alive, feel in control, and, what he had realised since, something about feeling superior as well, and, as he had uncovered in a following counselling session, the irony was he had been maintaining a gambling habit that, whilst it could make him feel that way, it could also leave him feeling like shit when he lost, when he didn't get that feeling he was chasing. At least he wasn't having to experience that any more. Yes, he'd realised that losing, not getting that feeling was also part of the experience as well, something else he had got used to, had become part of himself, part of his expectations. Yes, he was chasing the win, the good feeling that came from engaging in the gambling, the anticipation, the focus, the feeling alive, and there was part of him that in some way also fed off the loss, the come down, the day after, the feelings of depression that could also be present.

He felt he wanted to review things with Clive, in particular in relation to this other side of the experience.

Counselling session 12: exploring experiences associated with gambling

Max had sat down in the counselling room and Clive had asked him how he was and how he wanted to use the time.

'I've just been thinking, out there in the waiting room, thinking back to that session where I felt so energised, when I really got in touch with the stuff about chasing that satisfaction, and how I needed a certain level of "feel-good" to be satisfied. Since then, I've been aware of it, but not as sharply. I feel like I've done well in many ways, but maybe not as well as I'd hoped. I mean, I'm playing the computer games, as you know, and I'm not sure whether that's the answer. I think I'd sort of felt a couple of months back that I needed a really different lifestyle, really different. But it hasn't really happened. I'm at the gym three or four nights a week, and it's positive that I've maintained that, but I can find myself heading off early to play the games. And that's not good.'

'Mhmm, doesn't feel so good knowing that you are feeling that way.'

'No, no, it doesn't. I have to, I don't know, I mean, at least I am out more evenings now, but it's like maybe the initial enthusiasm is wearing thin?'

Clive nodded, he understood what Max was saying. 'So although you are out more, somehow you feel your motivation is, as you say, wearing thin.'

'I feel kind of caught between allowing myself . . .' He paused. What was he allowing himself? He'd lost his train of thought. Lost motivation, yes, but he'd still lost what he was going to say. 'Sorry, lost my train of thought there.'

'Mhmm, you were saying about being out more in the evenings but you weren't feeling the same enthusiasm.' Clive thought that maybe a recap on what he had been saying might help.

'Yes, yes, that's it, caught between needing to go out and yet wanting to be back indoors.'

'So there's a kind of tension between going out and staying in?'

'But I know I need to go out sometimes. I mean, not all the time, and maybe I'm overdoing it. I mean, I'm out at work and with people there, it's not as though I'm a recluse or anything like that. Maybe I need a bit of my own space but the difficulty is I immediately fill that space up, well, not always but enough to concern me, I fill that time with computer games.'

'So, it's about time for you and getting a balance that meets your needs.'

Max nodded. 'And about what I do with the "time for me".'

'Sure, you want time for you but you're not so sure about using that time for computer games.'

'No, and that's what I need to address. It's strange, the other thing I was thinking about just now, before coming in, was the stuff we talked about when I was saying about how losing, or not feeling satisfied by the gambling, can affect me.'

'Feeling low, depressed, if I remember correctly.' Clive could remember that exploration. It had highlighted to him the complexity of breaking an addictive pattern.

'That's right, and I can feel that way now when I think about how I may be sliding back into a pattern of getting hooked back on to the computer. It's like I want to play the games and win, get that buzz, that feeling, and yet, well, I don't always get it and I'm thinking the next day how much time I spent on it. And often it leaves me feeling tired, and that doesn't help.'

'So, two reasons for feeling low, not getting the experience you want every time you play, and losing sleep because of it.'

'Which happened with the gambling, of course. It's like there's another side to this. I mean, I find it too easy to stay up into the night, but I regret it the next day. And then the next night comes and it's, you know, I'll just play for a little while. But it isn't a little while. I set the alarm to remind me, but once I've turned that off, well, it's, ten more minutes, but it isn't, it's longer.'

'So, even though the alarm clock reminds you it's time to stop, you give yourself a reason to keep going.'

'I can't give myself ten more minutes. I need to be more aware of the time and make myself stop when I plan to, or think I plan to.'

'Mhmm, you want to be able to be ready to stop when the alarm sounds?'

'I have to. I know I have to. I've got to be more disciplined. But what I wanted to say was, you know, about the experience of feeling low, beating myself up about it, which I can do. I mean, when I used to gamble and lose heavily I felt awful the next day, and it was only the thought that it would be different next time, and the anticipation, that sort of pulled me around. I can really see that. I really can.' Max paused momentarily before continuing. 'But it's almost like I sort of expect to feel low, it's almost as though I need to give myself that hard time, not because I deserve it, I mean, I probably do, but as an experience in itself. It's like part of me really needs to feel like shit. And that's, I don't know, I'm sort of more aware of that at the moment. Not that the games make me feel shit like the gambling did, but it's like I'd sort of broken free of that for a while but now it's sort of coming back as I find myself uncomfortable with the time I'm spending gaming.'

'Sort of made you more aware of it as it re-emerges?'

'And it's like part of me wants that. It's familiar, part of the old pattern. I don't know, I can't really get hold of it completely, but it's like, yes, I need to feel alive, and I need to feel crap as well.'

'Like the feeling of being alive and of feeling crap are both needs that you have to satisfy?'

'Mmm, yes, and, of course, the gambling did that. And, OK, I've been focusing on ways of ensuring I can feel alive other than gambling, and that's fine, but there's this other need as well, and it's like maybe, just maybe, I haven't thought this through, but the time I'm gaming is allowing me to feel that way again, not as much, but perhaps enough, I don't know.' Max felt quite focused as he spoke. There was something about this topic that energised him, which was strange as he was focusing on something that had quite the opposite effect.

'So, the downside to the gaming, the feelings you are left with, say, next day, seem to be themselves meeting a need.'

'A need to feel bad about myself.' Max took a deep breath. He was feeling distinctly uncomfortable all of a sudden.

'As if you need to give yourself the experience of feeling bad about yourself.'

A fresh insight has been uncovered following a flow of empathic responding to what the client has been saying. The client has identified a part of his nature that he hadn't really grasped before, and it is inducing feelings of discomfort in him as his self-concept is challenged by this emergence. It is a difficult time for the client as he now has to wrestle with the insight and try to integrate it into his sense of who he is. It is important that the counsellor remains both empathic and can experience and communicate unconditional positive regard to that aspect of the client's nature that is emerging into awareness. The client is, in effect, moving towards an opportunity for fuller congruence. The counsellor must himself be congruently integrated into the therapeutic relationship. Otherwise the new insight may get distorted by some unhelpful response from the counsellor, and either submerge again or be integrated into awareness in an incongruent manner.

Max nodded, aware that he was feeling suddenly very hot, 'yes'. Clive stayed with his focus on Max, and with the thought of his need to feel bad about himself. Another of those moments was occurring, Clive felt, a significant moment. Something was happening. He felt the silence intensely, his own senses sharpened as he waited for what was going to emerge next. That was how he felt, as though he was waiting for something inevitable to happen.

Max, meanwhile, had closed his eyes. He didn't want to feel bad, he hated feeling bad, he didn't want that. He wanted to feel good. That was all he wanted, to feel good. Was that too much to ask? Was it? He felt himself becoming increasingly emotional.

'I-I don't want to feel bad. I just want to feel good, feel normal. I want to feel happy. I don't want to feel like I have to beat myself up because of what I do.'

'Yeah, you want to feel good, happy, normal; not feel bad, not beat yourself up for what you do.'

Max shook his head slowly. He felt his stomach, well, more his solar plexus knotting up. 'He didn't want me. That's what he'd said, he didn't want me.'

Clive guessed that Max was referring to his father, but he didn't want to jump in with that assumption. He kept his empathic response simple whilst remaining open to the sense of hurt that was emanating from Max.

'He didn't want you.'

Max was shaking his head. 'I wasn't what he wanted. I wasn't good enough for him.'

'You felt as though you weren't good enough for him.'

'I wasn't. He said he'd only married my mother because of me and, well, he didn't really care. I guess I wasn't what he wanted.'

Clive could see the pain on Max's face as he spoke. He was clearly fighting back his emotions. Max had opened his eyes and was looking down.

'These are painful thoughts for you, to feel that he didn't care, that you weren't what he wanted.'

'I suppose I never really felt any love from him. My mother, yes, she was there, she cared, but, I don't know, if I hadn't been born I guess both of their lives might have been better.'

Clive noted the switch that had taken place, from what had felt like a more child-like part of Max to a more adult reflection as he described how he thought things might have been had he not been born. It sounded so clear that Max had, and maybe still was, blaming himself. Should he voice that? Would he be making a connection for the client? He could see it, but was it within the client's awareness in those terms, just he simply hadn't voiced it?

There will be times when the counsellor will sense things that are present within the client's inner world that the client themselves have not sensed, or have not quite grasped hold of. It is a matter of professional judgement as to whether it is therapeutically appropriate for the counsellor to voice these things. This will depend on how pressing they feel, how connected

> the counsellor feels to the client when the experience emerges in their awareness, whether voicing them might direct the client away from a focus that they currently have and which is absorbing them.

Clive decided to stay with what Max was experiencing and communicating. He didn't want to direct him away from that. He reflected back what Max had said, whilst maintaining his warm acceptance of Max as a person in the midst of his painful remembering and experiencing.

'That's how it feels to you, if you hadn't been born their lives would have been better.'

'I shouldn't have been born. It was my fault that they weren't happy. I made them get married.'

Clive noted the switch back into the more childlike view of the events from Max's past.

'You made them get married?'

'Yes . . . , well, yes, I suppose I did.' Max felt himself shift as he was speaking. Yes, if he hadn't been born. But he hadn't asked to be born, had he?

Clive noted the hesitation and the frown now on Max's face.

'Makes you frown?' He sought to empathise with the facial expression as clearly there was something driving that change.

'Well, yes, I mean, I could feel myself just then feeling it was my fault. And in a way I guess it was. I guess that's how it must have seemed.'

'Must have seemed when you were a child?'

Max was nodding. 'Hmm. Yes, that's how I saw it, and saw it for a long time, I think.' Max felt strangely calm and quiet inside himself as he spoke. The emotions that had been present had now passed. He was left with a sense of how he had been, and yet somehow it didn't feel right to the way he was thinking now. Like he had two different experiences or views, yes, two views of what had happened. He looked up at Clive. It seemed to him that Clive was really there with him, somehow, like he wasn't so alone with what he was feeling, had felt. He'd been alone with it for so many years. 'I think I've always blamed myself.'

'Blamed yourself for how they were?'

Max nodded. 'I suppose you do when you're a kid. You blame yourself. The thought that if I hadn't been born, then they'd be happy.' He shook his head. 'Maybe, but maybe not. Who knows? Don't suppose they'd have got together, but you don't know, and I might still have been born, you know?'

'Mhmm, maybe.'

'Hmm. Maybe.' He took a deep breath and sighed. 'If I felt bad about being born, if I blamed myself for my parents not being happy . . . , I mean, that's how it seems. Is that possible?'

'You question it, feeling bad about being born and blaming yourself . . . ?'

'I think I do, did, no, maybe do. Maybe I still do.' He took another deep breath. 'And I guess I've always known it but somehow, right now, somehow it feels very present.'

'Like it's come more strongly into the present, into your awareness?'

Max nodded. 'Hmm. More to think about. More to make sense of.'

Clive, tight-lipped, nodded, feeling for the heaviness in the way that Max had just spoken. He voiced a response to Max's tone of voice.

'The way you say it, sounds heavy.'

'It is. Something else to deal with. Well, maybe I am dealing with it, talking about it.' He shook his head. 'Could that be why I feel a need to feel bad about myself? Is that really possible, all those years ago, still affecting me?' He was looking at Clive again, and to Clive it felt as though Max was seeking an answer to a question that he already had the answer to.

'A lot of years thinking that way . . . '

'Yeah, I guess I know that it can, it does, it has affected me. Like I have to kind of punish myself. Am I doing that? Am I punishing myself? I didn't start getting into gambling to do that, though. I'm sure it was about feeling good.'

'Wasn't something you thought about, you wanted to feel good, feel alive, and the slot-machines, the games gave you those experiences.'

The client has asked a series of questions, partly of the counsellor, partly of himself. The counsellor has not sought to give an answer but maintained empathy for the questions or for the feeling tone associated with the questioning. The questions do not need to be answered. These are natural questions as the client struggles to accept his new reality. Can it be so? Can it? Being allowed to keep his question unanswered the client is left free to draw his own conclusion and to integrate the experience in his own way without it being coloured by some 'clever' answer that an inexperienced person-centred counsellor might conjure up.

'Didn't make me feel bad. No reason for it to make me feel bad. We were having fun, enjoying ourselves.' Max was frowning again. It didn't seem to make sense, somehow. He hadn't beaten himself up as a child, not over his trips to the arcade. He raised his right hand, resting his chin in the palm, his other arm supporting his elbow, and sat back in the chair. He hadn't realised that he had been sitting so far forward.

'Mhmm, you were having fun, enjoying yourself, feeling alive in the amusement arcades.'

Max nodded, 'yes, yes, that's all it was. It was only later, when things were getting difficult, when I was losing money, that was when I started to feel bad. Don't know that even then I beat myself up. It was just one of those things, it happened, it would be better the next time. I didn't feel good about it, but I don't think I gave myself grief over it, no, that was later, I guess when I started to feel more uncomfortable about it, I suppose.'

'Mhmm, so, when you began to feel more uncomfortable with it, that was when you felt you started giving yourself a hard time?'

'Yes. So there was a time when I just felt, well, a bit depressed by it, and then, later on, I guess I felt more depressed and started giving myself a hard time as well, but I suppose throughout that time I was feeling bad about it, or feeling bad about myself, or something, I'm not sure, but I wasn't feeling good, that's for sure.'

'So, the way I'm hearing you is that to begin with you didn't feel loss or bad, that came along later, and the more you lost, the more uncomfortable you felt about the effects of your gambling, and the more you gave yourself a hard time.'

'And then, when I had a good run – which happened – then I didn't have those feelings.'

'Mhmm.'

'But my original question, what I was thinking about again earlier was my need to feel bad, to give myself a hard time, to, yes, to blame myself, the "it's your fault, now look what you've done". And, even as I say that, I know part of me was saying that it wasn't my fault, it was the cards, I was just unlucky. So I was fighting against taking any blame. And, yes, I know that's a real gambler's way of thinking. Everyone else to blame, never you.'

'So, the self-blame was a bit mixed. You sort of did and you didn't.'

'But it was there, and I certainly was feeling low, feeling depressed, I was bringing that on myself even though I wouldn't have admitted to it at the time. But I was. My question is whether that was deliberate? Were the lows part of what motivated me to gamble, and not just the highs? Was I kind of caught in a sort of, not sure if it's a catch 22, but it's certainly a double whammy, isn't it?'

'A double whammy of being driven by the need to chase the high and to experience the low.'

In fact, the addictive experience for many people is not double but triple: the actual addictive habit itself with all that is associated with that particular behaviour and the psychological high that may be the result and the psychological low that also may result. This is true not just for gambling, but for any addictive behaviour. People may chase a high but also be seeking the low that comes afterwards as they think about what has happened, or what they may have done under the influence, or simply the coming down phase from stimulant use. The gambler has the addictive habit of the gambling experience, the experience of highs on winning as well as the adrenaline and excitement within the gambling process, and then the lows associated with losing, or with the feeling when losses are later thought about.

'Maybe it came along later and, well, simply started to satisfy this other need in myself to blame myself, which maybe went back to . . . Is that really possible, I mean, all the way back to when I was born, or at least, when I suppose I started to feel responsible for my parents' problems?'

'Things can affect us, Max, over time. I think you're the best judge of what you feel from your past is affecting you in the present, or the recent past at any rate.'

'Hmm, well, I guess it'll still be around. I'm giving myself a hard time some days over the gaming.' He shook his head and sighed heavily, biting his upper lip as he did so. 'I've got to break free of this. Of course I wasn't to blame for my parent's stuff. I can hardly be said to be the cause of my own birth!'

'No.'

'But that's not how, I guess, I saw it. So, I need to watch that. It's something else that could cause me to relapse, I think. And, yes, not something I'd see as being such a threat but I can see how it could be if I really need to give myself that experience of feeling bad and beating myself up. It feels like something I need to remind myself of. Something to keep in mind when I'm gaming. Stopping when that alarm goes off isn't only because I need to stop to control it, but to avoid getting into a cycle of giving myself a hard time. And blaming, blaming myself, that's a big part of it.' He nodded his head thoughtfully.

'Yeah, blaming yourself.' Clive responded to the final focus in what Max had been saying, it felt like the first time he had really acknowledged that in those words quite so strongly, and acceptingly.

'So, something else.' Max was shaking his head again. 'I'm going to get through it, though.'

Clive noted how Max's voice changed as he spoke, he sounded determined. 'You sound quite determined as you say you're going to get through it.'

Given all the self-questioning and uncertainty as the client struggles with new insights about himself and what from his past has shaped and affected him, he has reached a point and a place in himself where he connects with his will to get through it all. And with this comes, as well, a sense of there being no way back. This is another crucial step upon the path of sustainable change. The client is working at freeing himself from patterns from his past that live on in his present. He is now determined to put a block on them rippling into his future. Is this not, in many ways, what counselling is concerned with? Assessing the present in the light of a more congruent experiencing of the past so that informed choices may be made as to what will be the most satisfying set of experiences upon which the journey into the future will be built. These may not be words associated with psychological processes, they may seem more philosophical, but human-beings are more than psychological process. The beauty and relevance of the person-centred approach is that theoretically it combines a philosophy of life with a psychological understanding of process. That is why it is so powerful and why it has such wide application, both within and external to the therapy room.

'I am. I think I'm learning all the time. Yes, I slip, lapse on something, lose some motivation and enthusiasm, but I know I can't go back.'

'Mhmm, no turning back.'

'No.' Max shook his head again. 'No. Can't go back. There's no future in going back. I know that, and I think more and more I am feeling that as well. Back to that head and heart split, or thoughts and feelings. Feelings are catching up now. I know I have to keep on keeping on, and I feel it as well. Yes, memories, experiences do tug at my feelings, do try and turn me around, as it were, but I can't let them. I can't. I can't risk it. There's too much to lose. OK, I don't know how things will work out, and, yes, I know that gambling, and to a lesser extent the gaming have given me a lot. They've been a big part of my life. They did help me cope, maybe, got me through some crap times. I've got to move on, keep changing, get some new experiences into my life. I know all of this, and, well, that's perhaps also where the feelings are hanging back a little. It feels scary, unknown, uncertain. Can't quite imagine what it will be like to not feel I'm a gambler. In a way I'm getting there with that, though I know it's early days. I hear that often enough at the meetings! But they're right. I've got a lifetime ahead of me, I need to take my time and make sure my life's what I want it to be, and not feel driven by the past. And that's it, isn't it? Being open to the present and to the future, and not being "past-dominated", as it were?' Max felt good as he was speaking. He felt as though he was recapturing those feelings from that previous session. He felt optimistic again, though maybe it was a more informed optimism. The session drew to a close.

Points for discussion

- What are your views with regard to the issues addressed in this session?
- How has Max changed in line with Rogers' seven stages of change and the Prochaska and DiClemente 'cycle of change' model?
- Evaluate Clive's effectiveness as a person-centred counsellor. How would you be different, and why?
- What have you gained from reading this fictitious account of therapy?
- If you were referred a client with issues similar to those of Max, do you feel your practice may have changed?
- How optimistic do you feel towards Max and what he is trying to achieve? What hurdles do you anticipate he has still to face?
- How do you react to the idea of counselling someone whilst they are getting support from another place, for instance, as in this case, through Gamblers Anonymous?
- Write notes for this session.

Reflections

Max left feeling positive and with a sense of purpose and direction. He felt as though he was more alive, somehow. He was sure it was because of those bottled up feelings, the self-blame, the guilt all muddled into his need to feel

good, and to feel bad. He was walking back to his car as he pondered on the
sessions he'd had with Clive. He certainly hadn't anticipated what he had
experienced, and yet it was what he needed, he could see that now, so clearly.
But he had to keep working at it, had to extend his horizons but not over-
stretch himself.

As he prepared to drive off he looked in the mirror to check what was behind.
So much of your life behind you, but you can't go forward only looking back-
wards. Somehow the thought was there in his head. Yes, I have to check behind
in case something is coming at me that I need to avoid or at least be mindful of.
He sat for a while longer pondering this. He could see the parallel. In a way his
therapy was sitting checking what was behind in readiness to move forward.
Well, he'd looked in that therapeutic mirror and yes, he'd seen a lot coming
from his past that he had to attend to. Now, though, he was much more
aware of what was happening behind him – had happened. Now he felt more
ready to drive off, to move forward, to move into the flow, into the future, whatever that would be. It felt exciting. As he turned on the ignition the tape he had
left in started. He'd forgotten about that. The guitar solo filled the car and filled
his head, so clear and sharp and full of emotion. He felt the goosebumps on his
back and neck. He sat and listened before starting the engine. He knew it would
energise him, such a powerful song. The vocals started, the wizard, so many
dying to build the tower of stone, the wizard from the top flies but falls and
dies, the question why, why did so many die? And then, that ending. His eyes
watered as he opened himself to the power of the words.

> Look, look, look, look, look at the tower of stone,
> I see a rainbow rising, there, on the horizon,
> and I'm coming home, I'm coming home.
> Time is standing still, give me back my will.[1]

He checked the mirror again. All clear. Time to move on. Time to build his own
tower of stone, his time had stood still for too long, caught in the gambling trap,
now he was being given back his will, now it was time for his past to die, time
for his own rainbow to rise on his horizon.

Clive was feeling very positive as well. He felt good about his work with Max. Yes,
it hadn't been easy, there had been lapses and uncertainties, and yet Max was
persevering – in his own way, and doing things that maybe some would say he
shouldn't do because they'd maintain his addictive behaviour, like the gaming.
But Max was doing what he needed to do, and he was sufficiently self-aware
to be able to acknowledge when he felt uncomfortable about something. For
Clive, one of the important aspects of person-centred working when helping
people with addictions was that you trusted them and kept the therapeutic
relationship alive. Yes, people could, and often did, lapse or relapse, but there

---

[1] From 'Stargazer', by Ritchie Blackmore/Ronnie James Dio, from the album Rainbow Rising
(1976). Published by Eule Music Inc./Armchair Music, BMI.

was invariably a reason and an opportunity for greater self-understanding to emerge. He felt convinced that there was an actualising tendency, that there was something about being a human-being – and he knew that Rogers talked of a more widely applicable formative tendency that operated throughout creation – something about being human that meant that there was this unseen push, trend – what was the point in seeking other words – actualising tendency did capture it.

So, trust the process, trust the client, accept and work with this tendency. Don't try and push it, don't try and make it take a particular direction, create the therapeutic environment and let it work its magic. Hmm, maybe that was going a bit too far. Or was it? No, it wasn't. That magic was there, a hidden potential. And no, it wasn't a gamble. It was a fact. Create the right quality of human relationship and people are likely to change constructively. That didn't mean that it was pain free, or that things might not feel worse before feeling better, or different. No one said that the path of constructive personality change was easy, or that it was a linear progression. People did have to go back and connect with bad experiences, painful events. Not always, but often. But that was how it was. And *he* couldn't decide when a client needed to address something specifically. It would happen when it happened and if the relational climate reflected person-centred principles and values, then he felt sure he could trust the timeliness of it.

So, now that he'd given himself a little pep talk, it was time to write his notes and get ready for the next client. No, he wasn't a gambler, he was a person-centred therapist, and he *knew* what he offered was a mix of science and art, and that it was therapeutically helpful.

PART 2

The betting habit

CHAPTER 6

Setting the scene

Rob watched the television viewer as the horse he had backed, Happy Lad, missed out by half a length. 'Shit.' He'd felt sure it was a winner. He shook his head, still looking at the screen, part of him refusing to believe that he had lost his money. He didn't always bet on the horses, he preferred the dogs, but, well, he'd been given this tip and he'd checked it with a mate who'd also thought it sounded worth going for. He felt someone pat him on the back. 'Never mind, Rob.' It was Jimmy. 'You were unlucky old son, probably didn't like running on the soft, been raining at Sandown all morning. But he put in a good effort, nearly got there, maybe another half furlong and he'd have got up. Jockey held him up too long, maybe. Left him too much to do.'

Rob heard him speak but it didn't give him much comfort. Another wage packet gone, or at least most of it. He'd get hell at home again. And it was his son's birthday coming up, they'd have to buy something on credit. Maybe he needed to get another card? Cards. Made it all too easy. In the old days he guessed people still borrowed, but maybe it was harder. He wasn't sure. He only knew what it was like now, today. He'd overdone it. But he'd felt so sure. So bloody sure. He turned, 'yeah, and maybe next time. Bloody hell, Jimmy, I'm running out of next times.'

'Yeah. Yeah. But, still, luck changes, I know. I've had good runs and bad runs. You're in a bad run, mate. It'll change, it always does.'

Counselling session 1: do I want help? Forming a relationship

It was three weeks later and Rob was walking up to the door of an organisation that offered counselling for gamblers, 'problem gamblers' were the words they used in their leaflet which they'd sent to his wife, who'd given it to him. It offered a free service. His wife had made it clear, either you do something about your gambling, or you're out. He'd got angry, wanted to hit her, slap her about, but his anger was more with himself. He was thinking back to that last bet on the horses – he'd stuck to the dogs since then, though not with that much success. At least he hadn't lost much and, well, he saw it as a hobby. Got him out the house a bit as well, and at the moment he needed that. She was giving him hell, and the nipper, well, he didn't seem to settle, always on the go, throwing himself about. Her threat to throw him out, well, part of him wanted it. Would give him a reason to go and then he could get on with his own life. And he knew that wasn't the answer as well. Yeah, they didn't get on too well at times, but he didn't want to leave, not really. He did care about Karen. OK, they fought at times, usually about his gambling, but there were good times too. They didn't seem to happen so often, though, these days.

The notice said, 'ring the bell and come in'. He rang the bell, he heard it somewhere in the distance. It was an old building. He went inside. At least it felt warmer than outside. It was bitter outside, first cold blast of the winter. He'd noticed it the last couple of days, working on the site. Bricklaying could be such a thankless task sometimes. He'd been glad to get out of school and get a job. Get a trade, that's what his father had always said. Yeah, well, he had, and it meant being out in the cold. Still, they had some laughs and a few beers at lunchtime and after work always helped. And he didn't just lay bricks, turned his hand to anything these days. Came with experience.

He noticed the reception hatch on his left and went over to it. 'Mr Cooper. I've got an appointment at 5.30.'

'Yes, please have a seat.'

He didn't have to wait long. He heard his name and looked up. 'Hi there, I'm Patrick, everyone calls me Pat. You must be Rob, Rob Cooper?'

'Yes, that's me, thanks.' Rob followed Pat to the counselling room.

'So, have a seat, whichever you like.'

Rob sat in the one facing the door. 'Thanks.'

'So, we had a chat on the phone last week and I talked about confidentiality and what we offer here and a bit about myself. Are there any questions? Just want to check that out in case there are.'

'No, no, it seemed fine. As I said, I've never had counselling before, so I wasn't too sure what to expect.'

'Can seem a bit strange, talking to a stranger and stuff but, well, see how it goes. So, where do you want to start?'

'Well, I'm here, as you know, 'cos of the betting. It's not been so good, you know? Been losing a lot, can't seem to turn it around. You get bad runs, like, but, well, this one's got bad and I've spent money I haven't got which hasn't helped. And it's making life difficult.'

'Mhmm, so the betting's a bit out of control and it's making life difficult?'

'Nah, not out of control, I can control it, just had a bad run, see. That's all.'

Pat nodded and had a distinct feeling that maybe what Rob was looking for was some betting tips rather than counselling. He voiced it, 'sounds like you need a few betting tips?'

'Come in handy, they would, but, well, it's affecting my marriage, yeah, and, well, I think I need to do something about it. Try and cut back a bit I guess. Not sure how. Don't really want to but, well, can't afford it at the moment, so I've got to do something. It was the wife, she'd heard about this place and said I ought to come along. Didn't want to but, well, she gave me a bit of an ear-bashing, know what I mean, and here I am. Keep the peace a bit, like.'

Pat has responded to the tone of what Rob is saying. The client is denying that he has a gambling problem, his only problem is his bad run. Pat has empathised with this because what he has said is an acknowledgement of this, even though no reference to it has been made. Yet it enables the client to disclose a little more. Perhaps Pat's response relaxed him a little, let him drop his guard. Clients can be quite guarded, particularly when they are not coming to counselling purely of their own volition.

'Mhmm, so your wife persuaded you to come, but you're not really too sure what you want to do about your betting.'

'It's like it's what I do, see, what I enjoy. I work hard, labouring and the like, and, well, I need to relax a bit and, well, the dogs have always been an attraction to me ever since I was a nipper. Used to go with my dad and, well, the track's only round the corner, easy to get to. So, three nights a week, that's where I am.'

'Three nights a week and been like that for a while?'

'Most of my life. It's what I do, what I enjoy. Yeah, atmosphere, you know, and meet up with my mates. Blokes I've known since I was a lad, grown up together. The missus knew that, she's from around the area as well. It wasn't a problem till I started losing, see, that's the problem. I need to stop losing, things'd be OK then.'

'Mhmm, OK, so as far as you're concerned, your betting's only a problem because you're losing. Otherwise, it's not a problem to you or your wife?'

'That's right. She's glad to have me out of the house, says I make the place look untidy. So I'm out of there. But, well, you can't just watch 'em runnin' round, you have to have a few bets, makes it a bit more exciting.'

'Mhmm, so you bet those three evenings when you get down to the track.'

'Ah, well, yes, and no. You see, I also go down the betting shop – or phone through my bets. Other tracks and, well, sometimes on the horses as well. Depends. And I've not been too lucky with them either just lately.'

'So, you're betting on the horses and the dogs, at the dog track and at the betting shop. And you're on a losing streak and it's causing problems at home, your wife persuading you to come here.'

'That's right. So, what do I do? What's the answer?' Rob sat back in the chair, waiting for Pat to tell him what to do.

The client has not come to counselling expecting to find his own answers. Whilst some clients view the counsellor as the expert who will tell them what to do, in this case there is a strong sense of challenge from the client.

He doesn't want to be there. His wife has persuaded him to come, or rather, issued an ultimatum, get help or get out. The counsellor must be sensitive to the attitude that the client is bringing into the counselling relationship.

'You want an answer from me, you want me to tell you what you need to do?'

'Well, you're the expert.' There was a note of sarcasm in Rob's voice. He didn't believe that Pat was going to help him. Anyway, he didn't want help, he was on a bad run and, yes, maybe Pat had been right earlier, what he really wanted was some good tips. But he didn't see much prospect of getting those here. He was wasting his time. But if he didn't come and the wife found out, well, he felt sure he could sweeten her up. He'd done it before, though she had seemed particularly adamant this last time. Anyway, he was waiting. So, what was this counsellor going to tell him to do?

'That how you see me, as an expert?'

'Well, you're the counsellor. You should have answers for people with problems like I have.'

'Mhmm, I should have the answer to your betting problem?'

Rob nodded. This counsellor knew nothing, wouldn't know one end of a dog from the other. Waste of time.

Pat was fully aware of the challenging nature of what Rob was saying and how he was being. For Pat this was a matter to be empathised with. 'You don't want to be here, do you?'

Rob hadn't expected that response, but it was nevertheless true. 'Yeah, well, I don't see how you can help me.' He remained sure of his belief that it was a waste of time but also slightly unsettled by the forthright way Pat had spoken.

'Mhmm, don't think there's anything I can offer you that will help you.'

'No, no, I don't. I mean, what do you know about the dogs, about betting?'

'Do you want me to describe the experience of betting, of winning and losing, different systems, how to judge form, where the tracks are, will any of this help you?'

'No, no, I don't suppose it will.'

'So my giving you information, or talking in the language of betting on the dogs, won't actually help you?'

'No, no it won't.'

'OK, so, I'm wondering what you want from me, from being here?' Pat well appreciated Rob's not wanting to be at counselling, wanting to be told what to do but feeling that he, Pat, wasn't someone who would have the answers he thought he was looking for. Although he didn't want to make comparisons, it was a familiar experience. Each client had their own take on it. He needed to empathise with Rob's experience and expectations.

Clients will push counsellors, test their credibility. Here, the counsellor is being empathic to this. Is he at risk of losing unconditional positive regard for the client? This depends on what Pat is feeling. Is he sitting full of

> irritation for a client who is with him but doesn't want to be there? Or can
> he accept that, yes, clients do sometimes find themselves pushed into coming
> to counselling, it's not what they want or where they want to be?

'You say it's confidential, right? So, if I didn't come, you couldn't tell the wife if
she phoned, I know she has the number and she'd do that.'
'We wouldn't say anything. We're confidential. That means we wouldn't even
confirm whether or not you are a client, let alone whether you are attending.'
'Serious?'
'Sure, people have a right to make their own choices in life. We're individuals,
we're adults here, able to make our own decisions.'
'So.' Rob thought about it. 'So, I wouldn't have to be here, would I?'
'No, if that's how you want to play it, that's entirely up to you, Rob. You OK with
me calling you Rob?'
'Yeah, sure. OK. So I could go now?'
'You could, do you want to go now?'
Rob shook his head. 'I could just walk out, yeah?'
'Course you could. I'm not here to stop you. It's your life, your choices, your call.'
Rob was curious. This wasn't what he'd expected. He'd at least thought Pat
would have tried to persuade him to stay. He felt another challenging response
coming on. 'You want me to go?'
'I hope you don't. I hope you stay and explore your betting and what you can
do about it, or whatever else you want to talk about.' Pat was being genuine in
his response. He didn't want Pat to leave. He wasn't indifferent. He appreciated
the difficulty some clients had in attending counselling, in exploring issues,
particularly when they didn't want to be there or didn't feel it would be of
any benefit.
'Hmm.' Rob sat and thought for a moment. 'I'll stay.'
'OK.' Pat didn't say 'great', it could have conveyed a conditional positive regard.
'So, what do you want to talk about?'
'I can talk about anything, yeah?'
'Sure, it's your time.'
'Hmm.' Rob stayed silent, unsure what to say. He felt awkward sitting there with
someone he didn't know, who seemed to not want to say anything except
in response to what he said himself. Didn't make for conversation. Didn't
feel right.
Pat stayed with the silence, he acknowledged to himself that it wasn't an easy
silence. He felt OK with it, accepting that Rob may well not know what to say,
or maybe how to say something. But he trusted that the process of being that
was present within Rob – maybe he should say the process of being that is
Rob – would lead him to say or do whatever he needed to do. And maybe
that was to be silent, though he felt sure that on the inside Rob was probably
far from silent. It was quite a step to come into counselling. His fantasy was
that Rob may never have experienced anything quite like this, it took some
getting used to. He knew a counselling interaction would be nothing like a

conversation on the building site, at a dog meeting, or anywhere else for that matter.

'Not sure what to say or where to start? It can seem strange having time to talk like this.'

'Doesn't seem right somehow. I mean, what do I say, where do I start?'

'Doesn't seem right to be here like this, not knowing what to say?'

'No. I mean, I'm here because the missus got in touch. She's been giving me a hard time.'

'Mhmm, she's been giving you grief, yeah?'

Rob nodded. 'She wants me to stop gambling. I can't do that. It's my life. Going to the dogs, that's what I do.'

'Mhmm, it feels like she wants you to stop something that is your life.'

'Yeah, it isn't going to happen.' He paused and shrugged. 'So what do I do?'

'What options have you got?' Pat thought about simply responding with 'what do you do?' but felt that actually, given the tentative nature of the counselling relationship, phrasing his response the way that he did would help to encourage the relationship. For Pat, this was a crucial factor. Without a therapeutic relationship, there was no counselling.

This is an interesting point. Person-centred therapy is very much a relational process, and for this to occur then relationship needs to develop between the client and counsellor. How much should the counsellor's responses, particularly in the early stages of contact, be influenced by this requirement? The counsellor has decided to focus the interaction. Is this unacceptably directive in the context of person-centred theory? Or is it expressive of an empathy for the situation, the stage in the counselling process as well as the client's question 'so what do I do?'.

'I'm not going to stop going to the dogs. That's for sure. And I don't want to lose my marriage. Yeah, we fight sometimes, who doesn't? But, well, we get on well too. Can't imagine being with anyone else. Known each other since we were at school. So, no, it's about losing money, that's the thing. It would be OK if I didn't keep losing. That's what I have to change.'

'OK, that sounds really clear. What you want to change, have to change, is the fact that you're losing money, and how much you're losing.'

'Yeah, so, I mean, maybe I need another system, I've thought about that but it's hard to change a system. What if just as you change it you start to miss the big wins? No, no, I need to stay with what I'm doing.'

'OK, so stay with everything that you're doing, is that what you mean, or with specific things?'

Rob thought about it. 'Well, I guess I lose more on the horses. I mean, yeah, and I've been betting more heavily recently, well, that's what's caused the problems.'

'So you've upped your stakes, then, on the horses?'

'Started a few months back, was getting a bit more money doing some extra work
during the summer and, well, I could afford to increase my stakes, yeah, but
now there's less work this time of year, hmm, but I'm still betting more than I
can afford. But that's how you win more, pay off some of the debts.'

'Mhmm, so by continuing to bet more you feel you can pay off the debts?'

'Yeah, but it doesn't happen.'

'Mhmm, so, what you're trying to achieve isn't happening?'

'Getting worse.'

'So, debts are increasing in spite of the amount you are gambling?'

Rob nodded. 'And then I had this really good tip a few weeks back. I was sure of it,
really sure. I really went for it on that one, and it lost. Bloody going changed
and, well, Happy Lad – what a name – anyway, just didn't have the legs, it
was coming up on the rail, another half furlong and he'd have got there, but
had too much to do, left it too late. That brought it all to a head. Lost a lot of
that week's wages. I was so fucking sure.'

'Sounds like you were really close.'

'Just under half a length. He was coming up but . . .' Rob took a deep breath and
sighed. 'And that's why I'm here.'

'That's what's caused you to be here.'

'Yeah. That's it.'

'So, the horses and the amount you're betting is the problem, more than the dogs,
is that right, is that how you see it?'

The client is now owning a need to make changes. The counsellor has maintained his empathy and perhaps the negative side of the gambling has
become more apparent to the client as a result, it is holding him on the fact
that it has produced problems.

'Maybe I should stick to the dogs. It's hard. It'd be really hard to say no when the
lads are thinking of a session. Really hard. I'd feel like, well, I mean, I couldn't
tell them why, that the missus is giving me grief, yeah?'

'Mhmm, couldn't do that.'

'Nah. But I need to cut back a bit, I mean, I know that.' Rob's thinking switched.
'Your leaflet, you talk about ''problem gamblers'', I mean, I don't see myself as
a problem gambler. That sounds heavy. OK, so I have some problems, but
they're not impossible, it's not like I can't sort them out.'

'Sure, though you have problems linked to your betting, it doesn't feel to you as
though you are what we call ''a problem gambler''.'

'Nah, not me. Just having a bad run and betting too much.'

'Yeah, that sums it up for you, a bad run and betting too much.'

'Yeah. Yeah, that's how it is.'

Rob lapsed into silence. It wasn't something that he didn't already know, but,
well, somehow it seemed more real to him as he sat there in the counselling
room. He had to get a grip on it. And there was that nagging voice around,

just one more bet, the next one will be the winner. Losing streaks can't last forever, hang in there old son, you'll get there, was the thought that was with him. And at the same time he was aware that he was beginning to doubt that as well.

Pat sat with Rob in the silence. To Pat, Rob looked lost in thought. It wasn't an awkward silence as the previous one had been. So he guessed that Rob was probably more openly in touch with what he was experiencing inside himself.

Awkward, anxious silences are generally expressive of incongruence, and frequently linked to where a client is experiencing something but is trying not to acknowledge it in awareness, or is aware of something but trying not to voice it in the session. Either way, a block on the accurate flow of communication is taking place. Incongruence is present. As this is one of the necessary and sufficient conditions for constructive personality change described by Rogers, it is therapeutically significant.

'You're not going to tell me what to do, are you?'

Pat shook his head. 'I rather think you know what you need to do, Rob.'

'Yeah, yeah, I do. I just don't want to do it.'

'Mhmm, yeah, know what to do but . . .'

'. . . but. I gotta cut back, I have to, don't I? I've over-stretched myself. Karen's right. We can't afford it. We've already got credit card debts we can only just cover the interest on. I just know that if I can get a little more lucky I can sort all that out.'

'Mhmm, so it kind of hinges on you getting a little bit more lucky. Would that sum it up?'

'Yeah, yeah. But I . . . Oh, I don't know.' Rob was feeling more aware of his mixed feelings about it all. Truth was, he didn't know what to do. And he was worried. He didn't want to get into more debt, that wasn't going to help. They'd talked about having another child, they both wanted that, a brother or sister for Harry.

'You don't know, but . . .' Pat empathised with Rob's struggle to say something and waited to see if he would be able to find the words for what he had begun to describe.

'We can't let the debts pile up. You read about people with these massive debts. You think, stupid idiots, getting themselves into that situation. But, well, I can see how it happens, and how it could happen to us. Yet I know I must start winning again soon. I mean, it's not that I don't have wins, I do, but nothing really significant, nothing big to make a real difference.

'So, you can see yourself heading for big debts if you don't change, though you still kind of hope that big win could be there for you.'

'It's there, just hasn't happened. And if I didn't bet on something that comes in, I'd feel gutted, you know?'

'Mhmm, knowing that would leave you really, really gutted.'

'Yeah. Don't want that.'

'So, you want to avoid risking that feeling?'

'Yeah, suppose I do. Yeah.' Rob shook his head. 'Yeah you're right, I do want to avoid that. Suppose that's why I keep betting.' He paused. An uncomfortable thought had come to mind. He didn't keep it to himself, somehow it felt easier to express himself to Pat, he didn't know why. He wasn't sitting there analysing it, just found it easier to say what he was thinking. 'Yeah, keep betting, keep chasing the big one. That's what I'm doing, chasing the big one, but how often does it happen?'

'I guess you can answer that with the people you know who are also betting.'

'Not often. But we all still bet, don't we? Yeah, some people seem luckier or maybe they just have more information, you know? There's some shady stuff that goes on, well, that's everywhere, isn't it? All about who you know and what you know. But I'm not in that league. Nah, I'm chasing, and I'm betting higher and I'm losing more. I've got to cut back. If I reduce the bets and maybe cut it out some days, or try to. I won't stop the dogs. That's too much part of my life. Not going to stop that. It's the other stuff I need to do something about.'

'Mhmm, so that sounds quite clear. Reduce your bets, cut back on the number of days you bet, see how you go.'

'Yeah, yeah.'

Pat had glanced at the clock and noticed the session was due to end soon.

'So, we've only a few minutes left today. Has it helped? I know you had mixed feelings about it all at the start.'

'Yeah. Yeah, it has. Helped me realise that the wife's right, I have to do something. Can't get into more debt. Can't keep chasing that win, can I, but it would just be the answer, so easy.'

'Mhmm, would be the simple answer to everything.'

'Like the lottery, yeah? Buy that each week and, well, can't not buy a ticket now, bit like my system, change it and if something comes up that you would have betted on . . . No, don't want that. No. Keep to my system with the dogs but ease back on the stakes and, yeah, try and cut back on the horses. I guess I knew all that but I'll give it a go.'

'Sounds a lot, yeah?'

'Yeah, feels like it. Just have to give it a go. Keep the missus happy.' He paused. 'Yeah, she's right. Sensible head on her shoulders, that woman. Fuck knows what she sees in me sometimes! Must have something she wants.' He smirked as he spoke.

Pat nodded and smiled slightly. Rob needed to assert his manhood. That was OK. End of a session, talking man-to-man about some difficult issues, and acknowledging his wife's role in forcing the issue was putting him under pressure. Maybe didn't want to be seen to be dominated by her, so he says what he just said. That's OK. It's part of him that needs to be heard.

In many ways Rob has said what might be deemed a typical male comment, or is that stereotyping men? Pat simply smiles slightly, and perhaps 'slightly' is the key word. It allows Rob's comment to be acknowledged. But Pat is choosing not to get involved in an exploration of this, it is the end of the session, Rob is perhaps re-establishing his persona for the 'outside world'. Had Rob made the comment earlier in a session a different response may have been more appropriate, possibly leading to Rob exploring at more depth what he thinks his wife sees in him and wants from him, and maybe he would go deeper into this and get beneath the comment he's just made.

However, there is an issue here to reflect on. Was Pat's response appropriate? Had Pat been a female counsellor and Rob had made the same comment, what would have then been the appropriate response at this stage in the counselling session?

'Yeah. And you want to come back next week? Is this helpful?'
'Yeah, yeah, I'll give it a go, see what happens.'
The session drew to a close and Rob left. Pat sat back in his chair reflecting on the session, and also aware of how smoky the room seemed. Rob was obviously a heavy smoker, though he hadn't asked if he could smoke. Some clients did. He could appreciate Rob's mixed feelings about it all. Would he have much success making changes? One session of counselling, he might make a few changes, but some would be harder, and some would slide away from him over time, perhaps. But he did seem to be more motivated by the end of the session. He'd come up with his own general ideas as to what to try and do. He's clearly not giving up the dogs, he's going to hold on to them. Well, yes, you don't change really important parts of your lifestyle just like that. A thought struck him. He wondered whether Karen, his wife, went to the dog meetings? He'd sort of assumed not, but then, well, maybe she did. He didn't know. He didn't need to know. He wasn't taking a formal history. The picture would build up over time, he was sure.

He felt it would be interesting to work with Rob. Clearly, he was at a stage in his gambling career at which things could now become significantly problematic, or he could choose to make changes to step back from possibly exacerbating the problems. It was time to rein it in if he could and if that was what he wanted. Was his betting satisfying other needs, or was it simply a habit, something you just did, part of the social fabric of where you lived? Was it a class thing, going to the dogs? He wasn't sure how helpful that kind of speculation was. It could lead people to make generalised statements that could have little bearing to a particular individual's lifestyle choices. No, he'd see Rob next week, no doubt hear how he had got on, or whatever else may have happened, and take it from there.

Points for discussion

- Do you feel Rob changed during the course of the session? If so, how would you define that change?

- Two very different silences occurred during the session. What features characterise silences? What therapeutic importance and value do silences have?
- Evaluate Pat's effectiveness as a person-centred counsellor. How did he convey warm acceptance and empathy towards Rob?
- What part did the counsellor's congruence play in this opening session?
- How do you feel about Rob as a person and his gambling choices? Do you experience any reactions that might affect your ability to empathise with him, or to warmly accept him?
- Write notes for this session.

CHAPTER 7

Counselling session 2: a few wins, 'it's not a problem', and a confidentiality issue

Rob had sat down in the counselling room and waited for Pat to close the door. He had had a good week and was feeling pleased with himself.

'So, time perhaps to absorb last week's session, and no doubt things have happened during the week as well. What do you want to talk about today, Rob?'

'Been a good week, really has. Had a couple of wins and, well, best part of a grand.'

'Mhmm. You sound really pleased.'

'Yeah. And it was the horses mainly, though I won a bit more with the dogs on Thursday as well. So, yeah, maybe my problems aren't so bad after all.'

'So, those wins leave you feeling that your problems aren't so bad after all.' He smiled warmly, he could see how pleased Rob was, and perhaps a little bit relieved.

Pat stayed with Rob. He knew in himself there was a sense of yes, not so bad until the next losing streak. But that was his cynical side. He was pleased for Rob, it must have helped some of his financial worries. He wanted to ensure that Rob's feelings of pleasure were warmly accepted by him.

> In this situation a counsellor from another theoretical approach may have responded differently, pointing out something in relation to, say, whether it was helpful to have a win just as he felt he needed to make changes. Or the counsellor may have responded in a manner that reflected their own misgivings, of maybe even a judgemental attitude. Such responses are not person-centred. The client has had an experience and is telling the counsellor about it. The person-centred counsellor seeks to convey empathy for what the client is saying and experiencing and to offer warm acceptance so that the client can experience this reaction from the counsellor. Anything else will convey at best, conditional positive regard and at worse conditional negative regard.

'It feels good. I mean, I suppose it leaves me now wondering what to do. I told Karen and she, well, she said that's fine but it isn't like this every week, that I still needed to do something about my gambling. We ended up having a huge row about it and, well, things haven't been too good since. I don't know, she just isn't satisfied. I thought she'd be pleased. Well, she was, sort of, about having the extra cash, but then, well, she started off on a "don't think this means you can just carry on betting like you have been, you'll only start losing again". In fact, at one point she said that if all those wins do is encourage me to carry on then she'd rather I'd lost. She's so ungrateful.'

Pat could feel himself sympathising with Karen's view, but Rob was his client and it was Rob's frame of reference that needed to be accepted and empathised with.

'So it caused a row and it leaves you feeling she's so ungrateful?' Pat didn't repeat all that Rob had said, simply conveyed the last thing that Rob had said. Was he being selective? He didn't think so. Rob had talked himself to the point of mentioning how ungrateful he felt she was and so Pat felt it appropriate to empathise with that so that Rob could pick up his train of thought without being distracted away from it.

'Well, I mean, we needed that money. I gave her some of it for different things and we paid some towards one of the cards. At least that will bring the interest down a bit.'

'Mhmm, so you gave your wife some and used some of the money to address the debts.'

'Yeah. And kept some back for myself of course.'

'Mhmm, so you had a little extra as well.'

'Yeah, well, I did have.'

'Did have?'

'Yeah, well, had a bad run on Saturday. Lost what was left. But I was unlucky. I was so close. But, well . . .' Rob didn't say anymore. He didn't really want to get into talking about that. Preferred to think about the fact that he had won and that his losing streak was over, that maybe he could turn things around now.

'So close, but . . .'

'Aargh, bloody dog seemed to lose his grip on the bend, looked like he maybe got caught by the dog in front. Otherwise, he'd have been up for it, no doubt about it. So, you see, I can pick the winners, it's just that, well, things happen sometimes.' Rob felt genuinely pissed off about what had happened. It kind of soured his week watching what happened. He didn't want to dwell on it. This week would be better. He knew it would. Things were changing for him.

Whether the win had been large or small, it might still have been used by the client as a reason for questioning whether he had a problem and whether he needed to make changes. It indicates that the client is not really ready to make changes, at least the part of himself that was recognising this need in the previous session has now been submerged, as it were, by the re-emergence of the part that carries the belief that his gambling's OK and he doesn't need counselling to change because he doesn't need to change. He was just unlucky. He is bolstering his belief that he can pick winners, just happened to be unlucky on a particular occasion. He makes no mention of all the other races he will have betted on and lost.

What is significant in terms of person-centred practice is that the counsellor does not challenge what the client is saying. He warmly accepts the view that the client is putting forward. It is what the client is saying he thinks and feels. The counsellor's role is to let the client know that he has accurately heard and understood what he has said, and to maintain his unconditional positive regard. Other directive approaches would be more likely to challenge what the client is saying. But the client is not ready for that. If he was, he'd be challenging himself. Challenging clients can disrupt their structure of self before the internal processes within that structure have brought the structure to the point at which it naturally has to change under pressure from the working of the actualising tendency.

'Mhmm, so you're feeling more confident about your betting then this week?'

'Yeah. But she still wants me to come here. Still wants me to stop.' Rob shook his head. 'There's no pleasing her, know what I mean?'

'So your wife still wants you to attend and to stop betting ...'

'... yeah. Can't see it though.'

Rob had interrupted Pat before he had a chance to finish. He let go of what he was going to say and responded to what Rob had now said. 'Can't see yourself still attending here or stopping?' Pat wanted to clarify what Rob was saying as he was unsure and he didn't want to misunderstand him and maybe direct him one way or the other with a partial response.

'Can't see myself stopping. I don't mind coming here. Gets me out. It's OK chatting. Here, mind if I light up?' Rob was rummaging in his jacket pocket.

'This is a no-smoking building, so, no, that's how it is.'

'Getting more and more like that these days. Glad I don't work in an office or something. At least no one's gonna stop you smoking on a building site! Suppose they'll ban it in the bookies next!'

'Mhmm. Fewer places to smoke.'

'They just want to stop people having any pleasure, that's how it seems to me. Haven't they got something better to do than worrying over who's smoking and where. Bloody politicians.'

'You don't have much time for them?'

'Nah, they're only interested in feathering their own nests. How much time do they actually work in their offices? Swanning off, all these extra jobs, on company boards and stuff like that. They should bloody well clock in and be paid for the hours they work, like the rest of us. My taxes pay for that lot. If I go moonlighting, the tax man'll be after me. Or if I sneaked off site to do a bit of work on the side, the boss'd do his bloody nut. But they do that, all the ruddy time. They're paid to do a job and they should bloody well be there doing it. Not that it would probably make much difference. Perhaps we're better off without 'em meddling in everything.' Rob shook his head. He hadn't much time for politicians of any persuasion. Used to believe that some of them wanted to help people like himself, wanted to improve his lot in life, reduce his taxes, make sure people had decent wages and not just the people at the top.

'Fed up with politicians, better off without them, yeah?'

'They all go off in the summer for their holidays but the country still runs itself.' He stopped and sneered. 'No time for them.'

Pat was very aware that it had been Rob raising the issue of smoking that had taken the dialogue down this political path. He didn't want to direct Rob back, but he was also aware of what Rob had said about it being OK chatting. He wasn't offering a chat, but equally he knew that for some people that could be therapeutically helpful.

At what point does therapeutic dialogue become a chat? And, when it does, who is to make the judgement that it has ceased to be therapeutic or of therapeutic value? So long as the client is saying what they want to say and the counsellor is maintaining an empathic attitude and not being drawn into their own self-disclosures and losing their role and focus as a therapist, then it would seem that it is appropriate.

There is also the fact that for some clients, the very nature of counselling makes it difficult for them to relate to the counsellor. Not everyone has the same command of language, or is able to demonstrate what has been described as 'emotional literacy' – a rather judgemental term that can encourage a view that some people are not able to be clients. The reality is that a counsellor must be sensitive and responsive to their clients, whatever their capacity to express themselves through words. It is likely, however, that the therapeutic process will lead to increased emotional literacy as the client engages with their own feelings and finds their own language for communicating what they are experiencing. This, however, will not always be the case for everyone and the counsellor needs to be able to work with clients who have a limited vocabulary with which to express themselves.

'Mhmm.' Pat decided to simply offer a minimal response and allow Rob to take the focus in whatever direction he wanted.

Rob sat in silence for a moment or two, not knowing quite what to say next. He felt he'd said what he wanted to say about politicians. That had passed. His thoughts ranged across the situation he was in, sitting in this room with a counsellor. What was he playing at? Why was he here? He didn't need to be. He'd had a good week, the betting wasn't a problem. He'd got it sorted. Saturday was unlucky, it would be different this week. He was sure of it.

'You said last week that I didn't have to stay?'

'That's right. It's up to you. It's your time.'

'Well, I reckon there are people who probably need to see you more than I do, people with real problems, who're really losing it. And I don't want to waste your time.'

Pat noted the shift away from the earlier comment about it being OK chatting. Now it seemed Rob didn't want to chat.

'That how it feels, like there are other people worse than you so you're wasting my time being here?'

'Yeah, come on, you must see people with really big problems. Yeah, OK, we owe a bit, but I'll get that sorted. Things are going to be different now.' Rob felt genuine in what he was saying. He felt sure things would be different. He'd pushed any nagging doubt aside. He didn't just think it would be different, he wanted it to be different and he wasn't going to let himself think any other way.

'I really hope so, Rob, I really do.' Pat was genuine in what he said. He really did hope that things would be different for Rob. He waited to see what Rob would say or do next.

'And if my wife calls?'

Pat smiled. 'Come on, you don't want me to cover for you.'

'You said it was confidential.'

'Yes, it is, and we'll keep to that. But I'm simply highlighting that you're using that as cover, which is not the intention behind confidentiality.'

'So what do you suggest?'

'Tell your wife the truth?' Pat wondered whether he'd overstepped the person-centred mark with that response, and yet he also felt that what he was saying was utterly genuine and, yes, he didn't want confidentiality to be manipulated, but, yes, the service was confidential and he had a contract with his client to maintain it.

'You kidding?'

'Well, it's up to you. I'm sure you will do what you feel you need to do, Rob, on this one.'

'Hmm. It doesn't feel right telling her I'm coming here when I'm not, she's bound to find out somehow, probably have me followed one week. But if I tell her I'm not coming, well, she's still saying I've got to do something about the betting or I'm out. It was simpler before I came here.'

'Tough decisions, feels like it's more complicated now.'

'Rock and a hard place.'

'This place feel like a hard place?'

Rob shook his head. 'No, quite the opposite. Look, let me see how this week goes and, well, maybe discuss it next time. I mean, maybe I'll talk to her.' He stopped. He knew that wouldn't work. She'd been so vocal in what she'd said to him. 'This ain't easy, you know.'

'No, not easy at all.' Pat kept his empathy simple, not wishing to intrude in Rob's experiencing of his dilemma.

Rob did not want to come to counselling. He felt he was OK with his betting. But he didn't want his wife to know. 'OK, I'll come again next week. Don't suppose it'll do any harm. Gets me out of the house, like I've said. Gives me a

break from getting another ear-bashing. I can tell you about how well I've
done next week.'

'Sure, that's fine by me.'

'OK, well, look, I'm going to head off. Got to see a man about a dog.'

Pat smiled.

'It's true. I have actually, a contact who knows a bit of form. So, I expect things'll
be good again next week.'

'OK. So, you're heading off now, and same time next week?'

'Yeah, yeah that'll be fine.'

'OK. So, see you then.'

With that Rob left, looking at his watch. He had plenty of time, he'd arranged the
meeting on the assumption he'd be at the counselling for longer. Felt good to be
out of it. He'd see about next week.

Supervision: supervisee questions his congruence

'So, you said you wanted to talk about one of your new gambling clients, Pat?'
Ken sat with an air of expectation. He'd been supervising Pat for a couple of
years now, and he really found himself intrigued by the work Pat was doing
with his clients with gambling problems. He hadn't supervised anyone working
in that area before, and he had to say that he'd learned a lot. He had experience
of working with clients with addictions of other kinds and he was aware that
many of the issues and the ways of thinking mapped across, but at the same
time he recognised the individuality of each client. So, he thought, a new
client, and immediately wondered what fresh angle on problem gambling
might emerge from their exploration.

Pat nodded. 'Yes, his name's Rob. He's in his late twenties, married, young child,
works in the building industry, bets mainly at greyhound racing but also on the
horses. He's been pressured to come by his wife – and I think reasonably so
from her perspective. He'd lost a lot of money one week, they've also got debts
and I think she's basically had enough. And it was, as he said, a case of go and
do something about it or you're out. She sounds quite strong, given the way
Rob refers to her. Anyway, she's given him an ultimatum, and he's coming to
counselling.'

'But somewhat reluctantly.'

'Yes, very much so. I mean, last session, well, let me come back to that. The first
session, yes, quite reluctant at the start, expecting me to have answers, quite
challenging really. Got a sense that he was sort of testing me out. Was I going
to help him? I think in that session, or during that session, he accepted more
that he had a problem and needed to sort it out. I tried to not get ahead of him,
but stay with what he was experiencing and expressing. But he did get to a
point of planning some changes. Not too specific, more general ideas about

reducing the amount he stakes, and cutting down on trips to the betting shop, that kind of thing. But he did seem to be ready to give it a go.'

'So, from arriving not wanting to be there, he left with ideas for making changes?'

'I think so, but I also sensed that there was part of him that was accepting of what his wife was saying. I think he could see it had become a problem but, well, it's such a part of his life. Going to the dogs is something it seems he was brought up on. Went with his father and now he's carrying on the family tradition.' Pat paused. 'Don't know if his father's still alive, maybe he still goes with him. He never mentioned that. I don't know. Might make it a harder habit to break. But, you know, I can't see him changing that. I really can't. Or maybe I'm just picking up on how he feels about it because I know people change. I've seen it, people changing their whole lifestyle to break up a gambling pattern that's got out of control. But I don't know with Rob. I'm not sure how authentic he is.'

'Interesting comment, not sure how authentic he is.'

'Well, he's kind of wriggling, bit like a worm on a hook, I suppose. That's maybe the wrong image. He talked about being between a rock and a hard place. I remember asking if counselling felt like that – was that what I said? – can't remember exactly how I put it. Should have asked if that was what it felt like, but can't remember if I used the word ''felt''. Anyway, he said no, but it all came up around his being there because of what his wife was saying. She'd got our leaflet and given it to him, by the way.'

'OK, so she's very much the reason for him attending?'

'Yes, and what happened in the last session – our second – was that Rob wanted to stop coming and sort of hide his tracks through our confidentiality. In other words, ''you can't disclose whether or not I'm here, so I don't have to be here but you can't tell her that if she calls''.'

Ken nodded. 'Sounds familiar. You've had that before I seem to remember.'

'Yes. And we do hold our confidentiality. But there are people who try to use it and, well, I took the line of highlighting what I felt was happening, that he was using confidentiality for a purpose for which it was not intended, whilst saying as well that we would keep it nevertheless.'

'How did that feel for you?'

'It felt alright. I was saying it as it was. I wasn't trying to make him feel anything. My motive felt to me quite clear. I remember we'd talked all this through before in relation to another client.'

'Yes, yes, I remember.'

'So I felt I was being congruent in the relationship. It was a hard thing for Rob to hear . . .'

'. . . Hence the rock and the hard place.'

Pat nodded, taking a deep breath as he did so. 'So, I felt as if I was right to say what I did. Yes, we will hold confidentiality. Of course, there are limits to that and I'd explained that on the phone to him when we were arranging a first appointment. He didn't have any questions about it at the start of the first session. But there's a certain spirit to confidentiality, isn't there? And, well, I believe we have to be congruent to that as well.'

> The notion of a certain 'spirit to confidentiality' to which the counsellor needs to be congruent is an intriguing one. Confidentiality is there to ensure that a client attending for counselling, and the matters they are discussing, are kept confidential within the boundaries of confidentiality that have been agreed. But what of the client who seeks to use confidentiality in the way that Rob has suggested? In a way, we could see Rob's behaviour as a form of acting out which, itself, he has every right to be kept confidential. Perhaps the use of confidentiality as a deceit reflects other behaviours that are part of a client's established way of being. He or she will have every right to express those behaviours, and for them to be contained and boundaried within the counselling.

'Mhmm, congruent to the spirit of confidentiality, at least insofar as what we say, but the bottom line is that nevertheless the confidentiality is maintained.'

'But I felt that to be clear and congruent in myself I needed to voice my experience of what was happening.'

'Mhmm, and I can go with that. You sought to maintain clarity and transparency. Seems to me that it must have been quite a significant exchange between you.'

'It was. And, well, it then led me to say something about his having to decide what he wanted to do. That as far as I was concerned he could stop coming. I didn't want him to feel he couldn't make that choice, but I suppose what was present for me was the sense of the responsibility that comes with making that choice.' Pat paused for a moment. 'Hmm.'

'Hmm?' Ken responded with an inquisitive tone.

'Well, he asked about what options he had, something like that and I said, I think I said, though the words may not be accurate, something like, "you could tell your wife".' Somehow that seemed rather sharp as he spoke the words. And immediately that he had done so he remembered that this wasn't what he had said. And what he had said was actually sharper still. 'Ohh, no, those weren't my words, I've remembered them now. I said, "why not tell your wife the truth".' He winced again. 'He'd asked what his options were and rather than simply empathising with that, I gave him one.'

'You sure did.' Ken paused. He could understand how something like that could get said, but was it therapeutically helpful and where had it come from in Pat? What had stopped Pat from simply responding along the lines of, "you're wondering what your options are here". 'OK, you don't look too comfortable with that.'

'No, at the time it felt right, and I'm sure that's because I was being congruent to a part of me that was reacting to Rob. But that's not an excuse, just what I think happened. You can't judge whether a congruent response is appropriate just because it feels right.'

'No, no you can't.'

'Hmm, so, I guess it came from me feeling that I didn't want to be manipulated. All the stuff about confidentiality and what it felt to me, at least it feels this way now and I think it did then, that I was being drawn into a collusion. And I didn't want that. I didn't feel comfortable with that. It wasn't clean. It wasn't clear.'

'Mhmm, and you held your transparency and out came this response.'

'Yeah, but he could ... Yes, I know. I know it wasn't helpful. Kind of thing to notice myself feeling at the time and then say it here later, or after the client's gone or something. And, and yet there also feels as though there is something genuine and honest in what I said.'

'And sometimes it can be, and I don't want us to get into a right or wrong debate on all of this. It happened, let's make sense of it. Let's use it as an opportunity for greater understanding.'

'Thanks for that. I appreciate it. I don't feel judged, not by you, but when I was wincing just now I was certainly judging myself.'

'And that has to happen as well, sometimes, yes?'

Pat nodded. 'OK, so he hooked me. He drew out a response from me that was probably, more than probably, most certainly linked to feeling drawn into his manipulation of the meaning of confidentiality. I guess, in simple terms, I kind of retaliated. A sort of "you make me uncomfortable, I'll make you feel uncomfortable back".' Pat didn't like what he had just said, but he could see it, and it seemed so clear and obvious sitting here talking about it. He was so grateful that the climate of relationship in his supervision session with Ken left him feeling able to be open like this.

This comes back to the importance of the collaborative nature of the supervisory relationship. Something happens in a session. It isn't about then blaming the counsellor for what has happened, but about creating an opportunity to explore, make sense of, understand, and where necessary through a process of enhancing the counsellor/supervisee's congruence, ensuring that if it was unhelpful the likelihood of it happening again is minimised. That may seem a rather convoluted sentence, but to say that to ensure it doesn't happen again is unrealistic, particularly when something may have happened for the first time. You cannot guarantee that. Counsellors are human-beings and can have off days like everyone else, and are unlikely to maintain perfect empathy, congruence and unconditional positive regard for 60 minutes in every therapeutic hour. Another client, maybe with a slightly different focus, could draw out a similar though different reaction, and that would then also need to be explored. However, should it keep happening then clearly there will be an issue requiring further and perhaps more in-depth therapeutic work.

'Mhmm, that how it seems now, reflecting on the process?'

Pat nodded. 'Something about Rob had got to me in a way that I think I missed. He set up a reaction in me – and that sounds like I'm blaming him and I'm not. Maybe I should rephrase this. I reacted to him in a way which I was unaware of.

So, I was incongruent, but so in touch with the reaction that I thought I was being congruent. Oh God, that's a minefield, caught being congruent to my incongruent experiencing.'

'Mhmm, yes, hence why congruence is so important and so difficult. We can feel so utterly sure of ourselves, sometimes, and maybe it is that very sureness that should warn us that perhaps we're actually not allowing ourselves to be open to questioning.'

'I wasn't thinking, it just came out. Felt a bit sharp as soon as I'd said it, but at the time of saying it, in those seconds before I'd stopped speaking, it seemed exactly what needed to be said.'

'Yes, exactly what needed to be said.'

'That part of me judged it as being needed to be said. But to my agenda. Hmm.'

'So, where does that leave us, you, me?'

'Leaves me realising I need to self-monitor more closely with this client though not to the point that I get self-absorbed, of course. And my reaction to feeling manipulated was very strong, wasn't it. I need to watch that. And yet, working in this area I've never felt it quite like that.'

'Mhmm, so there's something different about your experience of working with this client, with Rob?'

'There must be. But I don't know what it is. He doesn't know what he wants. He's swinging from thinking he may have a bit of a problem to having no problem at all. He'd had a couple of wins since the first session which had left him feeling he maybe didn't have such a problem after all, it was just a losing streak that he was now over. But then he'd lost some of his winnings again last Saturday, though he rationalised that as being just unlucky because the dog he'd bet on slipped or something on a bend, something happened, otherwise he felt sure he'd have won.' Pat took a deep breath. 'I don't know, maybe there's something about "I've heard it all before".'

'You spoke with quite a sigh there.'

Pat was being aware of what he was feeling. He felt tired, that was present.

'Maybe. Hmm.' He paused before continuing. 'Maybe I need a break.'

'You feel things are getting on top of you?'

'Perhaps. Maybe it's the time of year as well. The clocks have gone back now, haven't they, the darker evenings. I usually take a week off around now to give myself a boost, head off somewhere a bit sunnier. Maybe I should have done that this year. It's been a busy time.'

It is important that counsellors monitor their workload and themselves to detect overload. Months of working without a real break can build up. The supervisor also has a role in looking out for this. It can be helpful for the supervisor to every now and then check whether a counsellor is having breaks. Offering counselling is exhausting. Counsellors may feel energised by the therapeutic work that they are doing, but it takes energy to maintain concentration, and re-creative time is an important element in maintaining their professional competence and psychological well-being.

> We might suggest that supervision, continuing professional development and regular re-creative activity together provide the personal and professional basis for healthy and productive counselling practice.

'Yes, I know from what you have been telling me. So maybe Rob has unwittingly flagged up for you that you need a break.'

'Maybe I should be grateful. But I still know I have to watch myself, and my reaction to him. There's something about him and, oh it's so easy to get stereotypical, and I don't want to do that, but he is. He's fairly slight, looks quite anxious at times like he half expects someone to jump out at him, you know? He doesn't look as if he could relax easily. I haven't thought about it much, that's how he is, but he does look like someone who bets on the dogs. And I know that's crazy and maybe I shouldn't think that way, but he does. And maybe that's because for Rob it really has become a way of life. I'm surprised he doesn't run dogs himself – maybe he does, he hasn't said anything about that, but I think maybe not. But he was brought up on it and it just feels like it's so much part of his life.'

'So, you don't want to be stereotypical in your description, but it's hard not to be because – let's use a psychological phrase – he's like a kind of archetypal "greyhound man"?'

'Yes. So maybe that's in part why I've reacted, I don't know. I just don't know, but it's something for me to consider. Maybe I'm seeing the stereotype and I'm reacting in a stereotypical way. You know, the more I'm thinking about this, the more I think maybe I've stumbled on to something here. Am I seeing Rob as Rob, or as some kind of melting pot of all greyhound fanciers, some composite person on whom my unresolved issues get dumped? God that sounds dramatic. It can't be as bad as that, but I wonder if that's not the flavour of it.'

'Mhmm. Sounds to you as though this has real meaning for the way you feel yourself reacting to Rob.'

'And yet, I haven't really thought like this in the sessions. I mean, it's like, yeah, I suppose I did notice some of these things, but they weren't issues, I didn't sort of dwell on them. But now, here, it's like, where was I?'

'Where were you?'

'With Rob, listening, but am I really so out of touch with myself?' Pat was noticing an edge of anxiety in his voice and within himself. 'Now I'm feeling anxious.'

'Mhmm, all this leaves you anxious about . . . ?'

'Am I messing up as a therapist?'

'And?'

'I don't know.'

'Mhmm, you don't know.' Ken tightened his lips. He didn't feel any doubt towards Pat. He experienced him as a highly competent professional and as a person who he related easily and well to.

Pat sat with his feelings. He shook his head. 'No, I think I've over-reacted. I know I do a good job, my clients do seem to benefit from and value the counselling I offer them. No, it's just that this does feel big.'

'And I want to acknowledge that I experience you as a highly competent counsellor, and I'm not doubting your ability. And these things happen, and we learn from them as best we can. And this feels particularly big.'

'You know I think I have some assumptions about gamblers, and they've built up in my mind over the years. There are certain traits that I witness time and time again. Yes, each person is different, but there are commonalities. And they're often similar to other addictive traits. Deviousness can be one of them, but I also know that people are devious for a reason, and often because something is happening that is making them uncomfortable. I know that. And I hate the word anyway because it is judgemental. People are maybe not always straight about things because they are trying to avoid what they perceive will happen if they are open about whatever it is. Take the drinker who says they haven't had a drink when they have. They're maybe trying to maintain a belief that they don't have a problem, or maybe they don't want the reaction they expect from others if they admit to it, or maybe they need to feel whatever they feel in those moments of denying they've had a drink, when they know that they have. Yes, denial's another one of those words that's so loaded with judgement.' He paused, 'anyway, getting back to Rob, maybe he's hooked some assumptions I have – I'm not even sure assumptions is the right word – anyway, whatever the right word is, a sensitive part of me, or maybe an overloaded part of me, has maybe reacted. I need to be aware of that and take steps to address that over-sensitive or overburdened part.' Pat felt better at having said all of that. He waited for Ken's response.

Working over a period of time with a particular client group does leave the counsellor recognising common traits, simply because they exist. This isn't to undermine the belief in the uniqueness of each individual. The difficulty then is that it can and invariably does mean that the counsellor builds up a kind of image and carries a degree of expectation as to what may be present for a particular client. We can't 'un-know' what we know. But the counsellor must be wary and ensure that the body of knowledge that he or she has collected in their own mind doesn't generate assumptions or influence their practice, for instance, affecting the quality and focus of the counsellor's empathy in such a way that client behaviours/thoughts/feelings that match the counsellor's expectations are acknowledged more and therefore encouraged as a focus.

'Overburdened or over-sensitive. Maybe they're hard to separate, each contributes to the other.'

'I think I need to find some quality time for myself, switch off, wind down. I need a bit more "re-creation" in my life, a bit more fun, have time out from the heavy stuff. I think I've let things get too narrow, too much focus on work and not enough play. Maybe I'm the one that needs to go to the dogs, loosen up a little.'

'That how it feels?'

'Well, I need to loosen up. Yes, it's been hectic and heavy going these past few months. I'll maybe get a weekend away, that would be a start, and plan a longer break as soon as seems reasonable.'

The session moved on to one other client. Pat felt tired by the end of the supervision session. The discussion had put him increasingly in touch with feeling tired, particularly the last client that he spoke of who had some really difficult problems and which Pat was aware that he found quite emotionally draining. Yes, he thought, I need something restorative. I need to look after my own well-being, I'd taken my eye off that particular ball.

Points for discussion

- What were your reactions to counselling session 2?
- How might you have responded from a person-centred perspective to Rob given his reluctance to want to acknowledge he has a problem?
- What are your thoughts about Rob leaving early, and for counselling to continue even though the client is making it clear he doesn't really want to be there?
- Should other issues have been covered in the supervision session?
- How did you find Ken's responses? Were they particularly facilitative, or not? Find examples of either.
- Write supervision notes for this session.

CHAPTER 8

Counselling session 3: the client's wife attends

Pat looked at the clock, there were five more minutes before his session with Rob was due to begin. He had been sitting pondering again on the supervision session, and the previous sessions with Rob. He felt that he would be able to be more accurately present, with clearer self-awareness after the supervision session. And his thoughts turned to wondering what Rob's week may have been like. More betting? More winning? More losing? How had his wife reacted? How would Rob react? So many unknowns, at least to him, but not to Rob. He has lived his week, I have not. Strange, he thought, how I can be sitting here and about to hear about something that has already happened and may perhaps have profoundly affected my client. They have lived their story for this week, and I have lived mine. I will soon learn Rob's story and how it has affected him, and until he tells me I know nothing. And when he tells me, he will only tell me what he wants me to hear. So much will go unsaid and unheard.

Somehow it felt as though last week's session had been crucial, well, he had also thought the previous one had been as well. Maybe every session has particular significance and sometimes we glimpse what it is at the time, sometimes on reflection, and sometimes we may never know what may have had particular meaning or significance for a client.

He took a deep breath and closed his eyes. He liked to close down his visual senses before seeing a client, seeking to focus himself and find some inner calm from which he might accurately register impressions from his clients – spoken or unspoken. He sat quietly, allowing the calmness to be present within him, and for his awareness to be embraced by it. He took a couple of deep breaths and opened his eyes, he glanced at the clock and noted that it was nearly time for the counselling session to begin. He went out to see if his client had arrived.

In fact, he had, and was sitting next to a woman that he did not know. 'Hello Rob, would you like to come through.'

'Hello. Er, Pat, this is my wife, Karen. We've been talking and, well, would it be OK if she comes in for the session?'

Pat turned to Karen. 'Hello Mrs Cooper, good to meet you.' He extended a hand which she took.

'I think it would be helpful if she came in. I think that maybe it would be good for her to maybe ask some questions.'

'Sure, if that's OK with you Rob. Is there anything you want to say before we begin, before your wife comes in, or are you OK with us all being together from the start?'

'From the start will be fine.'

'I'm just concerned about whether he's taking it seriously.' Pat noticed that although Karen threw a glance in Rob's direction as she spoke, there was a certain dismissive air to her voice.

'OK, well, let's go through.'

Should the counsellor agree to the client's wife coming into the session? The client is indicating that he is happy. It may be that he might say something else if he was in the counselling room alone with the counsellor. Perhaps Pat should have offered that first, and then invited Karen into the session once Rob had confirmed that he wished for this.

At the end of the day the counsellor makes a professional decision. As a person-centred counsellor he will seek the direction from his client. The client has indicated clearly that he has discussed it with his wife and he is happy for her to attend the session with him. Pat accepts this direction and must then decide what he feels he can appropriately offer to them both given that he only has a contract for one-to-one counselling with Rob.

Pat led the way, thinking to himself that this was one scenario that he hadn't expected, but this was how it was, Rob seemed to want Karen to be present so he'd go with it. But he was clear that he would say something to begin with to clarify exactly what was being requested of him, and also clarify confidentiality for them both as he wasn't going to start disclosing any of the content of sessions.

Pat opened the door and ushered them. 'I'll need to just get another chair, won't be a mo.' He left them briefly and removed a chair from the room next to his that wasn't being used. He walked into the counselling room with it. 'Please have a seat.' Pat put the new chair close to the chair that Rob sat in and they settled down.

'Right, so, thanks for coming along. I want to just say that what Rob's been talking about in our sessions will remain confidential. If he wants to tell you anything then, of course, that is his choice, but I am not at liberty to break confidentiality. And I guess the other thing is to really check out what you both want to get from this session. You've obviously been talking. I wouldn't be offering couple counselling, of course, but I can certainly try and answer any questions you might have, Karen.'

'Well, as you probably know, he's still betting and I need him to stop. We can't afford it. The money simply isn't there. And I've made it clear that he has to stop.'

'Mhmm, OK, and yes, I know that Rob is betting.'

'It's hard enough coping with the little one, but he's out so many evenings and, well, we're in debt. I have to look after all the bills, he's useless at that. So I'm the one having to make excuses why we can't pay, or having to cope with the final demands. I'm constantly juggling the money we have and, quite simply, there isn't enough whilst he keeps gambling it away. I really am at the end of my tether and I've told him, stop or out. I need to know where I am. I can't rely on him. I can't be sure week to week how much we'll have. I don't want to live like that. It has to stop.' As she spoke Pat noticed that Karen only once looked across at Rob, just after she had begun speaking.

'Feelings are running high and you've had enough, is that right?'

'Yes.' Karen sat back in the chair and folded her arms, still not looking at Rob.

Pat could feel the tension in the room. 'OK, so, I appreciate you telling me this, Karen, and I'm wondering what you both want to get out of being here today.'

'Well, we talked about it.'

'Not so much talked. You've spent the week down that betting shop again, I know you have, and you were at the dogs end of last week, *again*. You can't keep doing this. We can't afford it.'

'I won last week.'

Karen took a deep breath and sighed. 'Yes, I know, and I wish to God you hadn't. Maybe then you'd have realised that betting is not the answer. It's not going to pay the bills.' She had turned to Rob at this point and was clearly looking and feeling angry and frustrated.

'I paid off some of the debts, and there was money left over for other things.'

'Yes, and it went on other things, as you put it, necessities, things we have to have. And now it has gone, and we still have debts and you are still gambling.'

'I know, I know. So what do I do?'

'Give it up.'

'I can't just give it up. It's my social life.'

'What, in the betting shop at lunchtime, in the afternoon when you should be working?'

'Sometimes.'

'Sometimes! Huh!'

The counsellor has allowed his client and client's wife to bring their relationship into the session. He has listened to what has been taking place, registering the tone of the exchange and the content. Now he responds, acknowledging what he is experiencing from their exchange and acknowledging his own genuine feeling that he wants their presence to be helpful in some way. He offers a simple empathic statement towards each of them and offers his experience of what's happening between them.

'OK, I can see that things are difficult at the moment, and I guess I want to try and ensure that you both being here is helpful. I hear your anger, Karen, I hear your feeling of being unable to give it up, Rob. And it seems that you're both taking up positions and, in a sense, digging in, if I can put it that way, ready for the next battle.'

'It's always a battle.' Karen was speaking and looking at Pat. I never thought it would be like this. I mean, I've got nothing against people having a bet. I knew Rob liked a bet before I married him, and we used to go to the dog track together before little'un was born. Now, well, he still goes, and I'm stuck at home, 'cept when I can get someone to look after him in the evening. But I don't like to do that, not regularly anyway.'

'Mhmm, so you knew Rob liked a bet but you weren't expecting it to be like it is now.'

'No, it was OK to begin with, but he's spending money we haven't got, and I can't seem to get through to him. That's why I thought it might help if he came here. So I called and someone sent me your leaflet. But it isn't working, is it?'

'What I'm hearing, Karen, is that you believe or believed that coming here would mean that Rob would be able to stop betting, stop going to the dogs, and pretty quickly, yes?'

'Well, yes, I thought you'd be able to make him see sense.'

'OK, I appreciate what you are saying, but it isn't that simple, it never is. And I'm saying that not because I want to make excuses or anything like that, but people do find it hard to change ingrained habits – which is what this is.'

'Well, yes, I understand that. I mean, I suppose I didn't want or expect him to just stop, I wouldn't want him at home all the time, but it would be good to see a bit more of him. It's just the money, that's the real problem. We can't afford it, it's as simple as that.'

'And whilst I don't want to turn this into a couple counselling session, I do think it might be helpful to hear if there is anything you might want to say in response to what your wife has been saying, Rob.'

The counsellor has acknowledged Karen's concerns and has sought to openly and honestly respond, indicating the difficulty in changing established habits. He has then said he doesn't want to turn it into a couple counselling session and then promptly takes the role of a couple counsellor! This may be an expression of anxiety on the counsellor's part. He may not be used to couple work. He may be feeling pulled between allegiance to his client and wanting to respond to Karen's concerns. It seems that he is trying to give Rob a voice, and maybe therefore not trusting him to be able to say what he wants to say when he wants to say it. It is a difficult balance to achieve. How long should he have continued in a dialogue with Karen? The person-centred counsellor will seek to be open, seek to allow what needs to be said to be said, and will seek to be responsive to the changing relational dynamics in the room.

'It's something I look forward to doing, something I enjoy. Yes, OK, so the money's tight . . .'

'. . . the money's not there!'

Pat was about to comment but Rob continued. 'OK, so maybe I need to cut back. But I did have that win, you know.'

'Sweet Jesus, you keep going on about that win. That was last week. What about this week? Tell him what happened this week.'

Pat was feeling concerned, this was becoming a very 'Karen-centred' session and he could understand why, and maybe she did need to vent her feelings of frustration, and maybe he could facilitate it in such a way that perhaps it had a productive impact. The truth was, he felt torn. He felt for Karen, struggling to hold things together financially. And he felt for Rob, suddenly being pressured into giving up something that was such a big part of his life. And there they sat, the two of them, neither wanting to give way. Rob looked across at Pat as Karen finished speaking.

'I had an unlucky week.'

'Unlucky! Is that what you call it? Who's going to pay the phone bill that came in yesterday? Tell me, where's the money coming from for that?' She shook her head. 'I think you're getting worse.' She turned to Pat. 'Sorry, no disrespect to you.'

'No, no, that's your perception. No disrespect felt.'

'It's just that I so hoped this was going to help. I know I shout at him, and, well, maybe that doesn't help, but I get so angry and frustrated. I still love him, I wonder why sometimes, he causes me so much grief, but, oh, I don't know. What's the use?'

Pat nodded, 'you love him but you wonder what's the use?' Pat was aware he had slid into an empathic response and he didn't want this to become a counselling session for Karen with Rob observing.

'I do love him. I don't want to throw him out. I'd hate that. I just want him to see sense, change a little, make some effort. That's all, make some effort. Try and be a bit different. Be there a bit more. Help out more. Little things, anything.' Karen could feel her own emotions rising and her eyes filled with tears. She felt wretched. She didn't want to have to feel that she'd have to throw Rob out. Not that she was sure whether she could, anyway, if it came to it. She just wanted to scare him, show him how serious it was. She couldn't think of any other way. 'I want us to be different, am I asking too much?'

Pat responded to Karen and then looked across to Rob. 'You want things to be different between you, that's really clear, and it makes you quite emotional thinking about it.'

Karen sniffed and nodded, and took a tissue out of her handbag, dabbing at her eyes. 'I don't know what to do, I really don't.'

Pat looked across at Rob, wondering whether he would respond. If ever there was a moment screaming at him to respond, this was it.

A crucial moment. The counsellor stands back, present and attentive but allowing the space to be open, giving Rob the opportunity to respond, to express what is present for him in response to what Karen is feeling and communicating.

'I don't want to be thrown out, and maybe I'm not much good with money. I'll try harder, love. I don't want you upset. But it's not easy. I know you're sick of me mentioning that win, but ...'

Karen sighed loudly and visibly.

'... OK, OK, I know you wish it hadn't happened, but it did. And, well, maybe it encouraged me to bet more. Maybe I thought, and maybe it was a stupid thought, maybe I thought my luck had changed.'

'Do you ever see a poor bookmaker? Do you ever see betting shops closing down? No. They're always opening new ones, at least, that's how it seems. Why? Because there's money in it, yours and mine.'

'People do win. I've had wins in the past, you know that.'

'Yes, I do know that, but we can't afford to take the risk any more. We've got to get our finances sorted out. I'm not going to spend the rest of my life in debt, arguing with everyone over when they'll get their money. I've had to do that, but not forever. I want a different life to that. You talk to them. You tell them where the money's gone. See how well they take your, "well, I won last week".'

Rob shook his head. He'd had nothing but criticism about that win, and even he was now beginning to wish he hadn't had it as well. It had proved more trouble than it was worth. 'When are you going to stop going on about that win? I thought it was a good thing, maybe I should have said nothing and just kept the fucking money.' Rob had had enough. He didn't want to be there, he didn't want to hear Karen going on about it any more. He'd had enough. 'Seems to me that this is a total waste of time. You want me to stop something that I can't just stop, and that, to be honest, I don't *want* to stop.'

'If I heard Karen correctly, I thought she said that she'd wanted you to stop or else she'd throw you out because she wanted to shock you into changing.' Pat felt he wanted to clarify this as clearly part of the problem was the way they were both polarising at extremes. "Rob – I can't stop. Karen – you have to stop". Somehow, if there was to be any progress here, yes, the demands needed to be heard and understood but the actual end result would have to be a compromise.

Karen nodded. 'I accept you won't stop, but cut back and spend more time at home, that's what I'm really asking for, Rob. Don't you want to spend time with me any more, or with Harry?'

'Course I do.' He took a deep breath, feeling his own emotions suddenly becoming very present. And he could feel himself again wanting to say something about that win, but this time he bit it back. What good would it do going on about it, just made things worse. 'Yeah, course I do.'

It seems that they have both stepped away from their polarising positions and a point of agreement is being exchanged. Pat's interjection has enabled them to relate to each other through a common point of interest, being together, something deep down they both want but they keep losing sight of it in their polarised reactions. What is important is that those strong reactions are being aired, that they are being made visible and vocal. And whilst each may not feel accepting of what the other is saying, the counsellor's role is to ensure they are all equally accepted, if only by him. In fact, the dialogue hasn't offered much opportunity for this other than his remaining focused in his listening to both of them and not trying to stop either feeling the way that they do. He has simply sought to clarify what had seemed to be a definite misunderstanding on Rob's part.

'Can you forget about trying to make money by betting, just treat it as a bit of fun, not as some way to pay back debts? Just a bit of fun, and if you do win a bit extra, well, OK that'll maybe help a little. But maybe we can try and budget it a bit. I know you've been going to the dog track all your life, and how important that is. I know that. And I don't want to take that away from you. But you've got Harry to think about as well, now. It's not just you, or just you and me.'

Rob knew she was right. But he didn't feel comfortable with kids, never had. Felt awkward. Left it all to Karen. She was good at it. 'Yeah, I know. But I'm no good with kids, you know that.'

'Well, maybe we could try together. Maybe you'll be fine if you try.'

'Can't seem to relate to him.'

'I know, but he's your son, you're his father. He's going to need you. He's going to look up to you. What do you want him to see?'

Pat remained quiet but attentive and actively listening to the dialogue taking place between Karen and Rob. He believed that in a situation like this it was crucial that he remain focused. His presence was important, perhaps the one factor that was enabling them both to find moments of communication, periods when they could listen, when their emotions did not boil over and start causing the polarisation to occur once again. He made sure that whoever was speaking he gave full attention to and, when they finished, he would nod slightly and then look to the other person. He was not planning to say anything unless he felt something needed to be acknowledged that the other person was not acknowledging, or was showing signs of having not heard. It felt a bit like group facilitation – it was just a very small group.

Pat was also aware that with two people he was not only being given, if you like, two ways of being, two personhoods, he wasn't sure how best to think about it, but he was also being given that third factor, the relationship between them. They were living out their relationship in the room, the pain and hurt, the difficulty, the needs and the wants. He knew the session would end up as a kind of couple counselling session. But he knew, as well, that he needed to trust the process, all the processes that were combining into the one process of communication between Karen and Rob.

'Someone he can feel proud of. Someone he would feel good about being with.'

'I'd like that too.'

Rob swallowed. Now he was feeling emotional. 'I want us to work, love, I do. I'm not very good at it, though. I mean, I don't do feelings very well, you know that.'

'I know, but you can, I've seen you, felt your passion.'

'Yeah, well.' Rob suddenly felt uncomfortable. His thoughts had gone back to their honeymoon and then he remembered Pat sitting there. Well, he hadn't actually forgotten him, but somehow he felt uncomfortable having these feelings and thoughts with Pat around. 'Not something you talk about.'

'Not something we talk about much. We used to, though, didn't we? Driving out to the coast. Walking along the beach. Watching the sunset. We did those things.'

'It's what you do.' Rob was still uncomfortable, uncertain how Pat would react.

Pat could see through Rob's mannerisms that he had grown uneasy. He didn't want to rescue him, but he guessed that perhaps it was his presence as a man that might be causing the discomfort or unease, or whatever it was that Rob was experiencing.

'Seems like you've had some really tender moments, but they got lost somewhere but it's not too late to rediscover them.' Pat caught both their eyes and nodded slightly as he did so. He felt the atmosphere change. It was quieter now. The storm had passed, at least for now. Perhaps in the calmness something could be re-forged between them. He knew that one conversation wouldn't change everything, but perhaps they might leave working at Rob's betting problem together. That would be a powerful outcome for the session, if that was what they both wanted. But it wasn't for him to seek a goal for them. Time was passing. He glanced at the clock, fifteen minutes left. He decided to mention this so they were aware should they wish to focus on anything specific during the rest of the time. 'Fifteen minutes left, just so you are aware.'

'Thanks.' It was Karen who spoke. 'I came here feeling very angry. That seems to have lessened a bit. I know it isn't easy for Rob. I know we have to work at it together. It's no good me saying it's his problem, though I feel that way sometimes, particularly when things are difficult.' She took a deep breath. 'Problem is it feels like it's difficult more and more of the time.'

'Mhmm, feels difficult more and more of the time.' Pat empathised with what Karen had said, wanting not only to let her know that he had heard her, but also wanting to hold what she had said in the room. She had spoken in a way that sounded so heartfelt.

'I'll change. I know I have to. I guess I've not wanted to change, wanted to stay as I've always been. When you said about Harry and what I wanted him to see. That got to me. I don't want him to have a dad that's always in the betting shop. He'll end up like me. But I'd want to take him to the dogs.'

'That's OK, I don't mind that. It's something we can do together. I like going as well, you know that. We always went together.'

Rob was taking a deep breath. 'It's the betting, I've got to cut back. I've got to get it out of my head that I'm going to win, that betting's the answer to our problems. But it's so hard not to think that. I know I can win. I know it. But I don't win enough, do I? That's the reality. I don't win enough.'

'No, no you don't.'

'Hmm. It's hard to accept that betting's the problem when you've been thinking it'll be the solution. That's really hard.'

'Can't be easy. But you can see what I'm saying, can't you?'

Rob nodded. 'I know you're right, but part of me wants to fight against it, I know that. I suppose that's why it's a problem. Problem gambler. I remember saying here that I wasn't a problem gambler. But maybe I am, maybe I've got to accept that.'

'Problem gambler simply means someone whose gambling causes problems – to themselves or others.' Pat felt it appropriate to define this in the simplest terms.

'And if it wasn't causing problems I – we – wouldn't be sitting here now, would we?'

'Probably not.'

Rob took a deep breath and let it out. Karen reached over to him and took his hand. 'We've got to face this together, love, it's the only way.' Karen looked at him, her eyes were still very watery.

'Yeah, I know. I know.' Rob squeezed her hand.

Pat said nothing but allowed the moment of contact and connection to remain.

Again the counsellor keeps out of the way, allowing the two of them to relate to each other. He will not want to say or do anything to disturb the moment.

It was Karen who broke the silence. 'So, where do we go from here? What does Rob need to do?'

'Whatever Rob does need to do needs to be thought through and will need your agreement and support. I can't say what will be the best way forward, Rob knows what he feels most able to change, what will feel realistic. It may not be enough for you, not to begin with, but sometimes a slowly, slowly approach is more sustainable, but for other people they prefer a sudden and maybe more dramatic change. It comes down in part to personality. But what matters most, I think, is that whatever goal Rob sets himself, he has to own it and feel it is realistic. Does that make sense for you, Rob?'

The counsellor offers a view, an opinion. He is responding directly to Karen's question and is stepping away from his previously therapeutic focus as he facilitated the exchanges between Rob and Karen. Perhaps rather than facilitate we should say he allowed and witnessed their unfolding process. His role was to offer a therapeutic climate in which they could feel able to be with each other as they needed to be.

Rob nodded. 'I need to reduce the amount I bet, give myself a limit, cut back on the time in the betting shop and, yeah, spend more time at home. Maybe we should go out together sometimes as well. We don't seem to do that much either like we used to.'

'OK, now, you may slip on some of these things. What do you need from Karen, Rob?'

'Encouragement. If I slip up, giving me a hard time doesn't actually help. I know you get angry and frustrated, and you have things you want to say, but it doesn't always help.'

'And what do you need from Rob?'

'Honesty. I need to know what's happening. I'll try not to react if he bets too much and loses, I can't promise that, though. It's not easy. Sometimes I just want to explode.'

Rob nodded as he sat tight-lipped listening to what Karen was saying. 'It's because I think you'll explode that I keep quiet.'

'I'll try not to react, but I may do as well.'

'I guess we just have to do the best we can.'

'Keep the communication open. Keep talking if you can. Honesty is important from both of you, and it sounds like you'll both need encouragement from each other.'

Time was almost up. They both thanked Pat. Karen felt more at ease now and Rob felt more optimistic about his marriage, that maybe he could begin to make changes, make things a little better, a little easier at home. Rob asked Karen if she wanted to come for the next session but she said no, it was Rob's time but she might want to come again another time if that was OK?'

'Up to you both to discuss that. It's OK with me. If it helps you achieve what you want to, then it's fine by me.'

They both left and Pat returned to his seat. He realised how tired he was. He hadn't said a great deal but he had been concentrating hard throughout the session, listening to everything that was being said, trying to ensure that he was present, and experienced as a presence offering empathy and warm acceptance. He hoped his responses that he voiced had been helpful and appropriate. He felt as though they had been. Something had certainly shifted between Rob and Karen. Once Karen's anger and frustration had felt heard, perhaps? Maybe that helped her to be different which enabled Rob to be different, perhaps? At least they had moved away from the polarisation that so often caused such damage to relationships. He opened his file and wrote his notes for the session.

Points for discussion

- Was it appropriate for Karen to be allowed to attend the session?
- How would you have handled the start of the session? Would you have said anything different to Pat and, if so, why?
- What did you experience as you read the session? Were there times when you would have spoken when Pat was silent? If so, when, and why?

- What were the key moments in the session?
- One-off couple sessions may not always reach such a positive outcome. Consider the pros and cons of such sessions within a client's therapeutic process.
- Write notes for this session.

CHAPTER 9

Counselling session 4: struggling to accept the need to stop betting

The following week Rob was settling into the chair in the counselling room. The previous week's session had made an impression on both him and Karen, and they'd both begun to step back from the constant conflict that had been developing over recent weeks and months. He was still betting, but he was making efforts to limit it. And he was beginning to realise that one thing he was finding difficult was being seen not to bet in the same way as some of the other guys on the site. He was very conscious that he wasn't betting the amount that they were, at least those who were in the 'betting club'. It was something that was on his mind as Pat sat down and spoke.

'So, how do you want to use the time we have today?' Pat was deliberately not going to mention the previous week's session. He did not know whether Rob wanted to talk about that or not. He tried to be careful at the start of sessions to ensure that the client felt able to take their own direction, thereby keeping to the non-directive emphasis of person-centred working.

Rob sat quietly for a moment or two before speaking. 'Well, I'm cutting back a bit. Not betting so much. Trying not to think about it as being the answer to our financial problems, just trying to see it as a bit of fun. But it's not easy. It sort of feels too serious to be a bit of fun.'

'Serious?' Pat responded with a questioning tone, he was unsure what Rob meant by his use of the word. He wanted to be sure that he accurately understood what Rob was meaning.

'It's like, well, I mean, it is serious. It's not just a bit of fun, not for me or for the other guys. They're serious about winning, like I am. That's why you do it, to win. Not for fun. But I know I have to think differently about it, but that doesn't come easily.'

'So, it's like you're trying to think differently about it but actually that isn't the way you really feel about it?'

'I go down the betting shop to win, or when I place a bet at a meeting, again, it's to win. That's why you do it. Yes, I know it makes for excitement and all that, and maybe some people do it for that, but me, I'm looking to win. I want a return.

I can't help that, it's how I've always betted. I'm looking to make some spare cash. And, yeah, OK, we have a few laughs as well, but I'm there to make some money.' In fact, Rob wasn't sure whether anyone could be said to bet for the fun of it, did you need money on a dog to have fun? Yes, it sharpened it up a bit, course it did, same with the horses, but he just wanted to get some extra cash.

'So, your main motive is the money?'

'Yeah, I mean, that's what makes it a good feeling, you know? If I've lost, OK, I'll tell myself it'll be better next time, but I don't feel good about it. I can't say to myself, "oh well, you lost, but at least it was a bit of fun". I'm not there, that's not how it is.'

'Mhmm, betting for fun just isn't you, it's a serious attempt to make a bit of extra cash, and if you lose, you don't feel good.'

'I don't. And I suppose, OK, maybe if you're super rich and it doesn't really matter how much you lose, well, maybe then they might say it's a bit of fun. But I'm not there. I'm out to win. I take it seriously.'

'As you say, for you betting's a serious business, you want to win.' Pat continued to stay in contact with what Rob was saying. He clearly needed to be heard around his motive for betting, and that it was at odds with the idea of betting for fun.

'It's like a kind of, well, not exactly a job, but it's more than a hobby, yes?'

'Yes, somewhere between a hobby and a job.'

'And, yeah, of course I enjoy the social part, mainly the dogs that is, I'm not so sure about the betting on the horses any more. It's like I'm feeling like I maybe shouldn't be doing it. I don't know. It's weird. I haven't felt like that before.' Rob was genuinely concerned as he really was experiencing mixed feelings in the betting shop, and he hadn't felt that way at all at the dog meetings he'd been to since the last session.

'So the social side of the dog meetings feels the same, but the betting shop experience is sort of leaving you uncomfortable. Is that how it is?'

Rob nodded. 'It's like I'm sort of watching myself.' He shook his head and paused. 'After last week me and the missus, we had a chat about it and, well, we agreed that I'd limit what I bet, at least to try and make sure we don't add to our debts, at least that's a start. And she went through with me all the bills we had outstanding. I'd never really sat down and done that before, just left it to her to sort out. There were so many, guess I hadn't thought about it. I don't take cards with me to work, that's something we came up with, and I'm only taking a certain amount of cash. Feel a bit like a school kid with pocket money. But, well, I think it's the only way, for a time at least.'

'Sounds like you've both been working at it, coming up with ideas to limit the betting. But having sort of "spending money", is uncomfortable but it seems like a good idea – at least for now.'

'I guess I've got to get used to it if I'm going to change. But I can't see betting for fun working. I can't think differently about it. I bet to win, to get a return. OK, so I have to accept if I bet less I'll get less back. I'd rather think I could win more, but, yeah, I can see I can't take the risk of losing heavily. Maybe one day things'll be different, but that's not how it is now.' Rob had come to accept the reality of the situation. It didn't sit easily. He wanted to blame Karen, she'd not handled the money right. He'd wanted to blame the guys at work for encouraging him to bet more than he could afford. He wanted to blame the stupid horses that should have won, but didn't, or the dogs that he was so sure about that faded or never got in the frame. In fact, he'd wanted to blame anyone or anything except take responsibility himself. But now he was beginning to grasp that he played a part in it all as well.

The reaction of denying there's a problem, and if there is then it's someone or something else's fault is a common reaction where a habit of any kind has become problematic or to some degree addictive. Accepting responsibility for one's choices and decisions may not come easily. The person-centred counsellor will want to ensure that these thoughts and feelings are heard and understood. They are important feelings in the client. Yes, the counsellor may see them as 'excuses', but to the client they may be a genuinely felt belief, or they may be an attempt to deflect awareness from experiencing any sense of responsibility, as that might be too difficult to countenance.

Whilst some might argue that the counsellor is simply colluding with an unreal perspective, the unreality is centred in the counsellor's frame of reference. The client may not be experiencing this, and it is the client's frame of reference that is the focus for empathic listening and unconditional positive regard. As the therapeutic relationship develops, as trust is felt and the client begins to expose more of his or her inner world and experience, and realises that difficult areas can be expressed, which can bring a sense of relief and a lessening of anxiety, then the likelihood is that the client will eventually begin to own the choices and decisions that they have been making. This, however, cannot be pushed. If the counsellor attempted to point out to the client his or her incongruencies then the client who is not ready for this will deny or block, and could, in extreme cases, simply absent themselves from further counselling contact.

The person-centred counsellor offers the therapeutic conditions which enable the client to experience incongruencies rising into awareness, and offers opportunity for them to achieve greater congruence in their own self. Recognising the true causes of a gambling or betting habit, and the part that they have played and do play in maintaining the habit is a significant development. It is a sensitive process and must be undertaken at the client's pace and in collaboration with the client's internal psychological process.

'So, you are seeing it a little differently, having to accept that the price of losing less is that you may not win as much. And that's how it has to be for now.'

Rob took a deep breath, 'yeah'. He lapsed into silence. That had just about summed it up. What was getting to him was that he didn't feel so comfortable in the betting shop. He was now thinking about how much he could afford to bet, he hadn't thought that way before. It wasn't that he'd betted outrageous amounts in the past, there was a sort of natural limit, but now he was having to think about it, think about how much he'd bet on each race. It was taking something away from the whole experience. But he was determined to try and keep to a limit. He'd been tempted to borrow. Borrowing from your mate somehow seemed different. Wasn't like getting into debt, not the same. He wasn't sure why. Maybe with a mate, well, you knew you'd pay it back, that's what you did. But with a credit card, well, he'd got into the habit of not thinking about paying it back, well, just not thinking. Need another bet, put it on the card. Never crazy money, but it mounted up, he could see that now.

Pat sat with the silence, waiting to see what Rob wanted to say next. It felt a focused silence, not one full of anxiety or with a sense that the client was stuck with what to say. Rob looked thoughtful. Whatever his thoughts were Pat guessed that, for the moment at least, he needed to be with them.

Rob was still pondering about the betting shop. It was like part of him didn't sort of want to be there. No, that wasn't true, he wanted to be there and he wanted it to feel like it always did, but now it didn't somehow. Now it didn't. Just wasn't so satisfying, like there was always part of him having to think about the money. He resented it, he knew he did, having pocket money for Christ's sake. Yeah, part of him really did resent that and he could lose sight of the fact that it seemed so sensible at other times, a strategy to help him get it under control. Yeah.

Pat continued to wait. He stayed still, not wanting to move in a way that might disturb Rob's train of thought. It was one thing to remind a client you were there when you had a sense that perhaps contact was being diminished by whatever the client was experiencing, however, Rob simply looked deep in thought.

'What gets me is that I'm having to think about what I spend all the time. It's like I'm having to ration myself and to tell you the truth it's pissing me off.'

'Pissed off by having to think about what you can spend. You used the word "ration", that's what it's like?'

'Yeah, and rations are sort of basic, what you need to survive on. That's what it feels like, just enough money to survive on, no slack, nothing. Shit, I work hard and that's all I have to show for it. It ain't right, doesn't feel right, it's not how it should be. A grown man, for Christ's sake, it ain't natural, know what I mean?'

'Doesn't feel natural, not having any more money than what you're rationed, and because you're a grown man.'

'Yeah, I should be able to make my own choices, feel trusted, yeah, feel able to live my own life.'

'Mhmm.' Pat stayed with what Rob was saying. He could hear the part of Rob that wanted to justify having more money to, more than likely, go back to his previous pattern of betting. But he maintained his empathy for what Rob was feeling and saying. 'Make your own choices, feel trusted, live your own life, yeah, that would feel good?'

'Yeah. Yeah.' Rob shook his head. 'Yeah.' He snorted. 'Yeah, and I know what would happen. I like to think I could handle it, but I haven't have I? My track record isn't too good, is it? I'm not a good bet. Form's against me, yeah?'

'That how it feels, you're not a good bet for, what, being trusted with money in your pocket?' Pat wasn't sure if he'd strayed off the empathy by giving an example, although it seemed very much expressive of what Rob was struggling with even though he hadn't used those words. He felt it was a kind of contextual empathy, or at least, an empathic response that put what he was saying into context.

'Well, haven't done too well in the past. I mean, OK, maybe things are different now. I can see I need to change. Maybe I'm different. I don't know. I think I am. But I know I'm not a good bet. That's the problem I suppose. I'm not sure I'd put money on myself on this. And there's part of me that wants to, that thinks maybe that would motivate me.'

'Like you need the reward of winning, or rather you want winning to give you a reward, something like that?'

'I suppose so, yeah, I do want to feel rewarded. Feels like I'm giving something up, like I'm losing something as well, and I sort of want compensation as well.'

'So, a reward for winning and compensation for what you're losing.'

'Yeah.' Rob smiled. 'Sounds great if you can get it.' He was shaking his head again and had tightened his lips. 'I don't know. Changing habits, it's bloody difficult. You don't think it'll be. Just think, yeah, you can make changes if you need to. Well, yeah, I need to, I know that. I don't like it and in a way I don't want to have to. It's like I need to but don't want to, yeah?'

'Mhmm, like you know you have to change, but don't feel that you want to change.'

'Nah, but then I want the money problems solved and things to be better at home, you know?'

'Mhmm. Like you want the changes to happen but not go through this experience to get there?'

Whilst we have to recognise that all persons are unique with their own individual ways of being, with embedded habits for all different kinds of reasons, nevertheless there is a fairly common experience amongst people who start to realise they need to make changes but have mixed feelings about them. They can so often find themselves wanting pain-free change, wanting the results without having to go through the process. But the behaviour change is the final effect of an internal process. That is why the person-centred approach has a significant role to play in encouraging sustainable change. It's not that the person-centred counsellor has a goal of making a client change in a particular way, but they know that the presence of the necessary and sufficient conditions for constructive personality change mean that change is likely to occur. However, unless outer change – which in the context of habits and addictions is important – is underpinned by internal changes, then it is unlikely to be sustainable, or if it is sustained then it will be a constant struggle, in effect the person becoming stuck in the Prochaska and DiClemente 'maintenance phase', never truly exiting their process of change, never moving on from the presence of inner, psychological patterns that are connected to addictive behaviour (Prochaska and DiClemente, 1982).

'I want to feel in control. I want to be able to say to myself, yeah, think I'll put some money on a particular horse, or spend an afternoon in the betting shop and feel I'm not stretching myself, but I'm not having to think about what I can afford. I want to feel I can take it or leave it, but more the take it, if you see what I mean.'

'So, feel able to make the bets you want, when you want, without having to be concerned about the money you might lose.'

'That's right. And bet on a dog that I feel has got a real chance, yeah, give myself a real chance of winning. But what I've been doing is getting sloppy. Betting for the sake of it. Yeah, still taking it seriously, still out to win, but it's like you look at the runners and you think, OK, one of 'em'll win, and more than likely the favourite. I've got no reason to think otherwise. But, well, betting on a favourite isn't going to give you much return. So you look down the list, see something that has a bit of form, slightly better odds, and you go for it. But you didn't have to, see, you're betting because it's there. Everyone else you're with is going to bet on something, so you do, don't want to be left out, but you haven't really got a really good reason for that particular animal, yeah. You're not using your head.' He tapped himself on the side of his head. 'You need to be a bit canny. But when you lose, well, you want your money back, so you do back something in the next race. Now you're chasing. I've been thinking about this. It's being able to draw a line under each race and make a decision on the next race based only on the pros and cons of betting on something in that race. I know that. But it's so difficult to think that way when they're about to line up and you've just lost and there's a chance to at least get your money back and a bit more.'

'Sounds like you've been giving it a lot of thought.'

'I have. I'm no mug, not really, but I know it got out of control. I stopped thinking like I should. I had a long chat with my dad over the weekend. Told him about what's been happening. He said to me, "son, you've got to be one jump ahead. Don't chase after lost money, it affects your judgement. And he's right. And I've got to do that, but I get caught up in it all. And I can't seem to be able to not bet on each race. And that's the problem, there are races happening one after another, different meetings. That's why it's better to go the meeting, there are gaps between the races. Slows you down a bit.'

'So, betting at a meeting slows you down, gives you more time to think, do you mean?'

'I think I've just got to keep away from the betting shop. I know that's the answer but I hate the thought. And I can't see how it'll happen where I'm working.'

'So, where you are working stops you from keeping away from the betting shop?'

'We've got a bit of a club there, and it'd be kind of hard to break out of it. We slip off at lunchtime and after work, and phone a few bets through as well if we haven't had time. They don't seem to care so much, couple of 'em are single, don't know how the other two manage.'

'Mhmm.'

'I guess one good thing is we'll eventually move on from this site. It's right near a parade of shops – handy for grub but the betting shop's on the end nearest to where we're working. And I guess it's been more of a problem since I've been working there. Too much opportunity. It's all too easy. But if I want to stop I've got to tell the other guys that I'm out of it for a while.' He paused, taking a deep breath. 'That aint gonna be easy.'

'I'm sure it won't be easy to tell them you're not going to be in the betting circle any more.'

'And I know I've got to, I mean, realistically, I've got to put a brake on it. Yeah, I had that win, and, yeah, I guess I did go on about it a bit, and maybe it wasn't a good thing, maybe it did encourage me to carry on betting. Probably did. But it's just as hard stopping when you're losing. The next one might have been the one you'd have won on.' Another pause. 'I don't know. Sometimes I think I'd be better off stopping and not having to think about what might have happened. But you can't do that. You can't help wondering. Like lottery tickets, same thing, once you start, once you have your system, your numbers, it's not easy to stop. They've got you. And they've got me for that reason.'

The counsellor has not said much, his empathic responses have been straightforward, allowing the client to talk at length and for his train of thought to flow. All the time the client is connecting with the thoughts and feelings that motivate him to speak in the terms that he is. It is enabling that part of him that thinks about his betting, that is thinking about change and how to change, to be heard. Being warmly accepted helps the client to develop his thinking further and affirm to himself what he needs to do. The ideas are integrated into his way of thinking, strengthening that part of him that is focusing the urge to change.

The session continued with further exploration of the difficulty in making a change to his betting habit. However, the more Rob talked about it, and felt that somehow he wasn't alone with it, that Pat was really in there with him, he realised more and more that he had to keep out of the betting shop. The job he was on was going to last a few more months. He mentioned the idea of looking to work elsewhere, but the money was good. And, yes, he acknowledged that he was earning more, but the betting meant he ended up with less. But it was a big job, secure work and no, he wasn't going to change that.

The session drew to a close with Rob heading off with a renewed determination to try and keep out of the betting shop. Whilst he knew he needed to do this, he was very aware that part of him was reacting against it. It had felt uneasy to acknowledge this to Pat, like it was somehow making him anxious in some way. He wasn't at ease with himself, he knew that. He was torn, and probably more so now as a result of the counselling. And, yes, part of him wished that wasn't what he was experiencing, he'd like to turn the clock back a few weeks, it was somehow simpler then. But he knew he couldn't do that and, anyway, he'd have still wound up with the same problems eventually. No, he knew he had to change, but to do so because he wanted to. That was the hurdle. He still knew that deep down he didn't want to change.

For Pat the session had felt intense and he was feeling pleased that Rob was developing quite a lot of self-insight. He felt that was important. Clients could feel so much a victim of their internal processes, sometimes with a lack of real understanding of what was happening to them and why they were struggling with a particular issue. Rob was getting a clearer grasp of what he was battling against – himself, parts of himself – that wanted to cling to the way it was. He knew it wouldn't be an easy time for him, and would perhaps be more difficult as he became more aware of his inner tensions. As they came more clearly into awareness they would tend to provoke crisis, or at least points of crisis would seem to arise, in which the person was confronted with choices. That seemed to be part of the process. It wasn't simple and straightforward. OK, maybe a few people could change like that but it seemed that for most there was still a pull towards the way it was for some time. He knew he would need to be as fully available in the sessions as he could be for Rob as he faced up to the conflicting agendas within himself, and accepted that his betting nature may assert itself sometimes, and at other times perhaps the part of him that he was seeking to develop, that controlled his betting might come more to the fore. He felt respect for Rob, he wasn't embarking on an easy journey. And he thought of Karen and how important her support was likely to be.

Points for discussion

- Assess Pat's empathic responding during this session, and what significance it may have had for Rob's process.
- Has the session affected your perception of Rob and, if so, how might that impact on your empathy and unconditional positive regard towards him if he were your client?
- Are there issues from this session that you might wish to take to supervision?
- How would you describe what is happening internally for Rob in terms of person-centred theory? How would you describe the landscape of his inner self?
- How genuine do you feel Rob is in wanting to change his betting pattern?
- Write notes for this session.

CHAPTER 10

An update on progress

Rob attended the next two sessions. He found it hard to break the betting shop habit. He was cutting back on the amount he was betting and he told Pat how he was keeping within the limits that he and Karen had agreed. He still chaffed at having to have pocket money but also admitted that it did help and he had to accept it however much he felt himself reacting against it.

He again talked about how he was mixed in his thoughts and feelings about the changes he was undertaking. He was feeling that although he could perhaps settle into his current pattern, he was also still uncomfortable with it. He explored again how he felt torn, how difficult it was for him to say no to his mates at work. They'd already ribbed him about how he'd reduced what he was betting. He hadn't dared to tell them about the pocket money. He realised in one session that they weren't really friends, people he could trust with what he was trying to do. They were simply people he worked with. Most of his real friends he saw at the dog track and he had mentioned to a couple of them about cutting back. One had been really supportive and had been really encouraging. Said he understood how it could be and, yeah, how money could get tight. He was someone who didn't bet very much, who had it pretty much under control, a sort of social gambler was the phrase in Pat's mind as Rob had described him.

The other person that Rob had mentioned it to was anything but supportive. He was someone Rob had known since school, but who was a heavy better. He was all for encouraging Rob to continue, not to quit, that it brought benefits. As Rob listened to him he realised that he sounded just the way he would have spoken a few weeks back. Somehow it made a deep impression. He realised that he wasn't in that place. It was tempting to listen and take seriously what was being said, but actually he knew he couldn't, not really. He was in another place. He'd found that in one sense quite pleasing. But it was also quite shocking as he thought about how he had been and how, if he wasn't careful, he might end up again.

Rob attended the counselling each week. He was consistent in his attendance. In fact, he was finding it fascinating. He was learning about himself and he could then see other people differently as well. But he also felt that it was placing him apart from people that he'd felt close to in the past. That wasn't so easy.

He was due for his eighth counselling session and wanted to talk more about how he was feeling towards other people, and try again to get some idea about how to break free of the betting shop routine.

Counselling session 8: the client is calmer, more reflective

The session had already begun with Rob saying a little about his week. He was still struggling with the betting shop though he had maintained control over his betting, in fact, he had brought it down a little more, but he was still going in there.

'It's just part of the habit of work, I guess. I mean, I am betting less, there's no doubt about that. Karen would tell you that. And we're paying off some of the debts we – well, I, mounted up – and strangely enough I've actually won a bit as well. I think I'm being more careful, more thoughtful, less reckless. We talked about this, I know. I wasn't betting because I thought something would win, I'd begun betting in the hope that I'd win. There's a big difference, yeah?'

'Yes, I can see that.' Pat could grasp what he felt Rob was saying, but he checked it out nevertheless. 'You're saying that you're being more selective, only betting where you think something will win, not just betting in the hope of winning without any basis for it.'

'And I'm finding I can do that. I don't have to bet on every race – well, I never bet on every race, but a good few. I don't have to, particularly the races when I'm not there to watch them running. That's significant too. And I'm not getting involved in phone bets either. I seem to have been able to say no to that. So that's helped as well.' Rob felt generally pleased with how things were going.

'So, a number of changes which add up to you betting less and maybe having more winners?'

> This empathic summary leaves the client feeling understood and able to move on, now engaging with a feeling rather than simply talking about behaviour. The focus has deepened. This is the power of good empathy. The more the client feels heard, the less they need to repeat themselves and the greater the likelihood that they will engage more deeply with what underlies the subject they are talking about.

Rob nodded. 'Yeah. I'd got desperate, I can see that now, couldn't then. Just had to bet, had to. But I've sort of pulled back from that now. But I feel weird.'

'Feel weird?' Pat sought to encourage clarification as he wasn't sure exactly what feeling Rob was experiencing, what meaning he attributed to his use of the word "weird".

'It's like I've said before only more so now, it's like I sort of don't quite belong how I used to with the other guys. I'm not following their pattern the same. I feel like I'm sort of apart from them in some way. It's not that we're keeping apart, nothing like that, but I'm aware of being different. Like I said before when I talked to Pete at the dogs, hearing him speak and realising he's like I was, and how I could be again if I don't watch myself. So full of how good betting is, how you shouldn't see it as a problem, that it's a way of life and you win some, you lose some, but you can win more and you shouldn't be put off when you've had a bad run. All that stuff. That's what I'd have said, and not so long ago. And there's still part of me that believes it, even though I know it's crap.'

'So, you know it's crap but you can still feel that part of you believes it.'

'But I seem to have that under control as well. I feel like I've changed, and I'm still changing. Something inside me. I don't need to bet the same, yes, that's it, there isn't the same *need*. That was there in the past. I had to. I wanted to, but I had to. It was like, yeah, not sure how else to say it, just had to.'

'Had to place a bet, yeah?'

'Yeah, had to, no thought of not betting. Just did it. Now, though, like I've said before, now I think about it more. Now I can make a choice. In the past I couldn't, I didn't. And that was really confusing me to begin with but I think although, yeah, it feels weird, I'm getting used to it, and to accepting that I'm sort of different to the other guys now.' He stopped and thought about what he had said. 'Yeah, that's how it is, sort of different.'

'Mhmm, so you feel different and you can accept that more now.'

'I can. It's like when Karen comes out with me, it sort of feels more like old times somehow. We're getting on better. She's encouraging me to take an interest in things more at home, the bills and stuff. Yeah, it does my head in sometimes but, yeah, it's important stuff. I have to get to grips with it. I can work out odds and what I should get back on a win, no problem, but check a bank statement?' He shook his head. 'But I'm trying – Karen says very trying! But, you know, I'm giving it a go. And she's encouraging me to spend more time with Harry. And, yeah, that feels good. We sort of play. Karen's involved as well. Sort of gives me a bit of confidence. Felt awkward at first, still do, but now, well, that's feeling good too. I'm sort of happier at home. Don't feel I need to go out the same to sort of get away, know what I mean?'

'Mhmm, you're more comfortable with Harry, with being at home, it's maybe a more satisfying experience?' Pat was aware that Rob hadn't used the words "satisfying experience", but the way he was hearing Rob talk and his sense of what Rob's inner world was like now, meant that it felt appropriate. He didn't want to get ahead of him, but he accepted that there were times when a person-centred counsellor would point out something he felt to be present, maybe something the client hadn't voiced.

This is a bit of person-centred 'therapy speak'. However, it is an expression of something that the counsellor has sensed to be present within the inner world of experience of his client. Sometimes it is appropriate to point out something that is sensed by the counsellor that the client might hardly have glimpsed for themselves. But care is needed. The intention is not to get ahead of the client which can simply mean the counsellor ends up leading the client to what the counsellor is sensing. It is to be undertaken tentatively, an offering of a glimpse of something emerging from the shared experience of exploring the client's inner world. It must emerge from a place of deep or strong connection and contact between the counsellor and the client. And it is certainly not a licence to the counsellor to intellectualise and describe from his head, his own frame of reference, what he may be seeing. That is not empathy, and it is not something that a person-centred counsellor would engage in.

'Yeah, it is like that. I feel sort of calmer, more relaxed about things.'

Pat nodded. He'd noticed that Rob sat more calmly in the counselling sessions, that sort of anxious look and slightly jerky mannerism that had been around early on had lessened to the point of being virtually non-existent. He decided to offer his experience as well, it felt appropriate to do this and would offer encouragement for what Rob was feeling, and, of course, it was genuine and authentic. 'I'm aware that you look less anxious as well, you seem to be more relaxed now in these sessions.'

'Really. Well, I'm glad you've noticed. Karen's said the same. And my mate Kenny, yeah, he's been supportive and he said something similar as well, said I seemed to be a bit more laid back about things, not so tense. And he sees me at the dog track when I've got reasons to feel tense.' He shook his head. 'Bloody dog last week. Don't know what happened, think he was carrying an injury, certainly pulled up pretty sharp, I don't know, took off like a good 'un. Thought it was in the bag. Local dog as well. Most of the stadium probably had money on him. Coming off the bend his back legs went and that was that. Went lame maybe, I don't know exactly. They said it was an injury. He shouldn't have run him if he was carrying it, don't think he was, wouldn't have been any point. But it was like I just seemed to accept it.'

Pat was maintaining his empathy, listening to what Rob was saying and hearing the slightly surprised note in his voice. 'You sound surprised talking about how you accepted it.'

Another example of the counsellor responding to both tone and content, conveying that he has a fuller appreciation of what the client experienced than simply the fact of the acceptance. It conveys to the client the level of attentiveness of the counsellor. There is a direct empathy for the way the client feels as well as what he is saying. Feelings may then become more

> deeply engaged with, if that is what the client wishes to do. It is likely that he will, it is probably a pleasant feeling.

'I was.' He shrugged. 'So I'd lost, but then I didn't have so much on, that's how it is now. Didn't have so much to lose. And it was sort of, "OK, he's pulled up, happens occasionally", and I was able to watch the reactions around me. People were cursing and swearing, thumping the chair backs, it was uproar. And I was somehow watching, sort of grinning, I was. I don't know, it was like I found it almost amusing. I'm sure if I'd caught someone's eye with the expression on my face they'd have probably thumped me, I don't know.' Rob shrugged again. 'Weird stuff. It's like it's not so serious now as it was. I mean, I take it seriously, I don't just bet on anything, but somehow it isn't so serious any more.'

'While you take it seriously somehow the whole betting thing doesn't feel as serious, or you don't feel so serious. I don't think I'm getting that right.' Pat realised as he was into his sentence that he wasn't catching what Rob had said. He felt it best to be open, then he could offer Rob the opportunity to say it again so he could see if he could grasp his meaning at the second attempt.

'It's like each bet is serious, I mean, you know, I bet to win. Always have, always will. I don't just bet for a bit of fun. That's not me. It's serious. And yet somehow it isn't as well. I don't know, I don't know how else to explain it.'

'It sounds like you're pretty clear what you're experiencing, what you're feeling, it's just I'm struggling with how you're describing it. But it's something about the betting is serious and yet somehow you don't feel the same seriousness in general like you did before.'

> The person-centred counsellor will want to be authentic. Pat knows he hasn't really grasped what the client has said. There's no point in making a stab at an empathic response when you've maybe lost the plot. Better to say you're unsure and to offer what you think you've heard and therefore what your understanding is.

'Yeah, that's more like it, like I can step back from it as well. And I don't know if that's me, I've changed. Or maybe I'm not betting as much each time so not having so much to lose, maybe that's part of it. Or maybe my expectations are different. I'm not constantly seeking that big win that I have to have to get my money back or to pay off a debt, or something like that.'

'What I'm hearing, Rob, and I might have this wrong, but it's like winning isn't as important.'

Rob thought about it. Was that what it was? Was winning less important to him now? Maybe. He thought about it a little more. 'Maybe, but ...' He wasn't sure quite what the "but" was, but there definitely was a but in it. 'I still want to win, I bet to win, it is important and yet, yes, you're right, it's different. Maybe not as intense. I mean, when you stand to win quite a lot, well, yes that does make it more intense – win or lose. But, well, maybe again it's about not betting such high stakes, maybe. Or is it me? Am I feeling different about it all? I don't know. That's something to figure out, I guess.'

'Mhmm, yes, you're not sure, could be the amount you're betting each time, your expectation is different, you may be feeling different generally, could be a range of things . . .'

'Yeah, and I'll tell you what, and I'm almost surprised hearing myself say this, but it feels better this way.'

'Feels better the way you are experiencing it now?'

'What you said earlier. More satisfying. It's like, yeah, more satisfying, that's a good way of putting it. Not so intense. I mean, I used to like all that, probably still might I suppose if I could afford to bet higher, I don't now. Maybe one day I'll find out. But I'm sort of getting used to betting less and expecting less, and maybe having a quieter life at home as well. Maybe that's helping. Yeah. Life's not so frantic, rush, rush, rush. Can't be doing with it.'

'Can't be doing with rushing around.'

'Nah, what's the point? Maybe I'm maturing, getting older? Maybe spending more time with Harry and Karen has slowed me down a bit. Well, you can't rush a two year old, can you? They go at their own pace in everything. You can't rush them. Maybe that's rubbing off on me a bit?'

'That's how it feels, he's slowed you down, helped you get used to a different pace?'

'Yeah, yeah, more I think about it, yeah, makes sense, that. I can see that.'

'So, that's a big change, and you can see it, it makes sense.'

'Yeah, it does. He's always messing around with these wooden blocks. Loves 'em. You buy fancy toys and stuff and he plays with these blocks. Don't know what he's thinking, just likes playing with them. Got me playing with them as well. Maybe it's the bricklayer in me, I don't know, training him up early. He can help me on the site when he's a bit older. Get 'im carryin' a hod!' Rob grinned. 'They don't make those for children otherwise I could get him practising. Come in handy, that. Learn a trade!'

'Sign 'em up while they're still young, eh?'

'I wouldn't have talked like this a few months back, maybe even a few weeks back. And we're hoping for another now. Be good if he had a little brother to play with, but if it's a sister, well, that's OK too. Think I'd rather have another boy but, well, not like going to the shop and choosing!'

'I'm really struck by the way you're talking, you really sound so, I don't know what the word is – enthusiastic – about your son, about being with him, and that's not how you were. It's like, yes, it's like he's got you playing and, yes, I know what it is, for me I can see more sort of child-like qualities in you, somehow.'

Pat feels it is important to share his perception. He doesn't want to take Rob away from his focus, but equally he feels it is important to describe this difference that he has noted. It can be helpful to offer feedback like this, but again, it must be undertaken with care and forethought. The risk is that a particular aspect of the client gets valued more than another part. The person-centred counsellor seeks to offer an equal valuing to release the client to be able to freely choose how they want to be for their own reasons, to satisfy themselves, rather than to match some communicated expectation or condition of worth from an external source.

Pat was still thinking to himself. Yes, it could be Harry teaching his dad how to play. It makes him smile thinking about it. The deal was, you teach me how to play and I'll teach you how to carry a hod! The atmosphere felt quite light, and Pat wanted to respect that and stay with it, yet remain aware of his professional role as well and not get overly drawn into banter.

'Hmm, maybe, maybe. And that isn't to say I don't take things seriously, I do. I think my problem has been that I wasn't taking seriously things that I should have been.'

'Things you feel you should have taken seriously but didn't, that seems the problem.'

'It comes back down to taking responsibility, and, well, I've not done that, not really. I can see that now. Just went along doing what I wanted to do, doing what I'd always done, and not really thinking about anyone else. And now, well, now I don't feel so good about that. I'm trying to be different and, you know, people have seen a change in me. And I want to keep at it, you know, I really do.'

'Mhmm, I can hear in your voice how important it's become for you to maintain the changes.'

Rob's focus had shifted to his past. For some reason he was thinking of his own childhood. It had been OK, but he didn't remember playing very much. He guessed he must have done, he wasn't sure. He remembered having videos to watch, being taken out by his mum to the shops, and to the dog tracks. Yeah, he could remember the flat they lived in and his older sister. Always seemed to be making herself up. Still does.

'Just thinking back, there, to my childhood.'

'Mhmm.'

'I think I was a pretty selfish kid, you know. Had my own things. Didn't really want to share them. Funny, though, don't remember having a lot. Don't remember playing much but I guess we did. I remember we used to play football a lot outside, either below the flats or over at the park. Suppose I was too young to remember. And I guess I was older when we were out playing. That was the problem in those flats, you stayed in, played indoors, I suppose, but it wasn't very big. I remember friends round watching videos. Didn't have computer games, stuff like that, not till I was older anyway. Couldn't afford it, I suppose.'

'So, not many games and having to stay in the flat watching videos till you were older.'

'Mmm, that's what I can remember. I remember going to the dog tracks as a child, the noise, the lights, the excitement, I can remember that. Used to go out a lot.

They were good times.' Rob sat quietly, 'yeah, good times. It all seemed so much simpler then, I guess, except school. Didn't get on with that too well. Couldn't really get a grip on it. Didn't see the point, really. Knew I wanted to work outside. Thought of being in an office all day, that's not me. Didn't see much point in qualifications. Suppose I regret that a bit. Think I learned more arithmetic betting than I ever did at school. Funny that, but that's how it was.'

Pat had continued to listen carefully to what Rob was saying. He nodded slightly and responded with what he had heard. 'Something seemed simpler about those days though you didn't get on with school.'

'Yeah. Well, you know, you had it all done for you as a nipper.' He stopped as a thought came to mind quite strongly. 'Suppose I've always expected that in a way, letting Karen get on with the money and Harry and stuff. Wasn't a problem, till now. I need to change. It's just a difficult adjustment.' He paused again. 'Always wanted to win, though, something about winning, having to win. I remember as a kid on holiday, in the amusement arcade. I really wanted to win, that was all I cared about. Never mind what was happening, I wanted money back out of it. I guess I'm quite money orientated somehow, but not in a responsible way. But I wasn't like that at sport, not the same I suppose. Maybe because we didn't have a lot when I was a kid, maybe it made me sort of selfish, I don't know.'

Pat was very aware of the reflective way in which Rob was talking. He was sitting, quite calmly, looking quite relaxed, and it seemed like he was just letting his thoughts drift. In a sense, it was good to see. Such a contrast to the anxious and quite angular person that had started coming to counselling those weeks back. He had calmed down and now, here he was, letting his thoughts range back over his past, and making some truly insightful comments about the effect it had had on him. These were quite personal disclosures and he, Pat, needed to remain empathically sensitive both to what was being said and the way it was being said. Rob needed to be reflective and he knew he must allow that to continue for as long as he felt he needed it. It felt to Pat as though Rob was making connection within himself, for himself. But he wasn't going to comment on it, that would direct Rob's focus away from being reflective to thinking about his being reflective.

It is not necessarily appropriate to comment on how a client is being in the session. It can disturb the focus, take them away from it. The counsellor will need to note what they have recognised and, perhaps, it may have a place later in the session, but not at the time. Sometimes people need to use the counselling space for quiet reflection, to in effect drift into kind of 'free-fall' within themselves. It can be therapeutically important. It is an example of their own process running at its own gentle pace, taking the client to whatever bubbles into their awareness. Sometimes quite valuable insights can emerge which the client would be robbed of if the counsellor acted or spoke in any way that disturbed their process.

'Feels like not having a lot made you selfish.' Pat spoke fairly softly, wanting Rob to hear what he had heard, but not wanting to jog him away from his process.

'Didn't have many toys, and what we had, well, some of it anyway was from the charity shops. I can remember going to them. Sort of brought up on them in a way though there weren't so many in those days. And the catalogues, yeah, I remember them as well. Mum was always ordering stuff and I remember looking through them, just turning the pages. So many different things. Funny that. I can remember doing it. She doesn't do it any more, and Karen doesn't. Probably a good thing. Another way of getting into debt. I suppose Karen's parents didn't do it, don't think they did, so she doesn't. But I can remember them. And dad going on at her about things she'd ordered. Yeah, that's right, forgotten about that. Funny how you remember things.'

'Mhmm, memories just come back to you.'

'Christmas, aunts and uncles, grandparents coming round. We were like sardines in that flat, but everyone sort of squeezed in. I remember all that.'

'Everyone crammed into the flat at Christmas.'

'Yeah, good times. But not many kids. Funny that. At least, they were older, more my sister's age – she's six years older than me. Didn't really get on with them. They'd sort of play with me, though most of the time they were trying to make me do what I didn't want to do. Being a pain. I'd get upset and react to being pulled about by them. They'd all stand around telling me how sweet I was, what a lovely little face I had. He paused, before continuing, 'Didn't get on with my sister, well, how many boys do? Then, when I was older, she was into boys, an endless stream of boyfriends. I used to be around, get in the way, made a bit of money, paid off I guess, bribed to go away. Rotten little sod I was.' He grinned.

'Mhmm, so difficult relationship with your sister and her friends, but made some profit out of her boyfriends later.'

'Yeah.'

Pat had noticed that time was passing and there were only a few minutes of the session left. He felt reluctant to let Rob know, didn't want to jar him out of his reflective state, but he knew he needed to tell him.

'I don't want to take you away from your focus, but we've only a few minutes left.'

Rob nodded. It felt good just thinking back over the past. 'Yeah, need to come back to the present, get myself back home.' He looked at Pat. 'It's kind of good to reminisce. Don't often think of these things. Good to remember where you've been. Suppose it can help you make sense of where you've ended up!'

'Early stages in our journey through life may set a direction or a tone in some way.'

'I think they do. I mean, betting was in the family, the dogs were probably where I started to learn to be a selfish little git, not having much and wanting to hang on to what I had. And that winning, needing to win. We'd play games, I mean, you know cards for pennies and monopoly, things like that. Even then, I had to win. Funny, not at sport at school, that wasn't the same. But maybe it was the money, even if it was monopoly money.' Rob shook his head. 'Yeah, funny that.' Rob glanced at his watch. 'Yeah, time to go. OK. Thanks for that. Haven't talked so much about the betting but, well . . .'

'It's not always necessary.'

'No, feels good to chat like this. Thanks. See you next week.'

'Sure. See you then.'

Rob left, aware of still feeling in that sort of reflective place, still thinking about the past. He couldn't remember how he'd ended up thinking like this, something must have happened in that session, but he couldn't remember what. But it felt good, and that was important. Yeah, he'd head back home. He was looking forward to being at home. Yeah, he thought to himself, that wasn't how it was a little while back.

Pat was also in quite a reflective state as well. It had been a concentrated session, at least, he felt that he had been concentrating. Rob had talked a lot and he'd really needed to listen, to be there as a presence as Rob spoke. It had felt good the time in that more reflective place. Maybe he needed to have discovered that calmness to be able to do that? It felt important. Not that Rob was necessarily coming up with massive insights into his gambling. But that didn't matter. Rob's own process of being was taking him to where he needed to be. Pat trusted the presence of the actualising tendency, and accepted that at times you couldn't necessarily understand how it was working. You had to trust it, trust that the client, given freedom and the experience of being unconditionally accepted, would move to how they needed to be. And maybe it wasn't always the contact of what the client was reflecting on that mattered so much as the fact that they had entered into a reflective state. His job was to maintain the therapeutic conditions and not get in the way of how his client needed to experience and express himself.

He wondered how many more sessions they would have. He thought Rob was doing well. OK, he hadn't stopped betting, but was he realistically ever going to stop? He thought probably not. He was making changes, and he was changing in himself. He was, perhaps, re-integrating more into the family whereas maybe before he was distancing himself. So long as he and Karen were satisfied with the changes. He was concerned, though, that Rob was struggling to say no to his mates when they were heading off to the betting shop. But, given time, maybe he'd find his voice. However, whenever a person was finding it hard to say no to going betting then it did mean a doorway was open for it to become more problematic again. His thoughts turned to Rob's memory of getting money off his sister's boyfriends. He shook his head and smiled. Nothing changes, he thought, as he remembered the sweets he bought as a kid from the proceeds of being bought off by his sister's boyfriends.

Points for discussion

- What were the key moments in this session, and why?
- In what way do you feel the reflective phase of the session was important? What role do such periods have in therapy?
- What are the challenges that you feel now face Rob? Do you think he will ever stop betting? Should he even try to stop?

- Assess this session and all of the sessions with Rob in terms of the process of change that he has passed through. How would you describe that process in terms of person-centred theory?
- How do you feel about Pat's style of counselling? How would you describe it? What are his strengths and weaknesses as a person-centred counsellor?
- Write notes for this session.

CHAPTER 11

Pat reflects on his work with Rob

Pat's reflections – 'I'm enjoying working with Rob and am encouraged by the changes he has made. It's confirmed for me that clients have to want to change in order to change. He was very uncertain to begin with, and the win threw him back, but the session with Karen, his wife, seemed significant. I know that there are times when a spontaneous couple session can end up simply being another venue for the arguments to be repeated. In a sense, it was in their session, but I believe that by feeling heard and not judged, they were both able to move away from the polarising positions they were taking.

'There's no doubt that Rob did trigger off some stereotypical thoughts and feelings within me early on. That was my stuff and I had to deal with it. And now he's really challenging me. He is showing me a different side to his nature. The family man is emerging, developing, I'm not sure what word to use. And, yes, it is heartening to see that. I certainly didn't have that as a specific goal at the start. I knew I hoped he'd reduce the harm associated with his betting, but how he would achieve that and what changes would be required for him to achieve that, I couldn't be sure. He had to own his need to change, he had to begin to want to change as well, and that took time. Of course it did, he wasn't decided. At times he thought he was, then he swung back the other way. That's how it is when you begin to contemplate change. Yes, some people may wake up one morning and decide to change, but that decision is not in isolation. They will have passed through a phase before that of thinking about it, deliberating on it, maybe making a few attempts and sliding back.

'I feel good about my relationship with Rob. I look forward to our sessions. I find it encouraging to hear the way he is speaking. And I want to say as well that if he had not made the changes that he had, if he was still indecisive and perhaps being devious about his level of gambling, I would hope that I would warmly accept him and his need to be that way. That's the challenge of person-centred working – conveying warm acceptance to the whole person, and not being selective. Part of Rob knew he needed to change, another part didn't want to change. We can think of them as distinct parts, or simply as regions within his structure of self that overlap to some degree. At the end of the day, Rob wants to feel good. He wants to feel he is winning. He likes to feel in control.

He's realising that there is more to life than betting. He's finding other ways to feel good, to get a satisfying experience – at home, with his son, betting less and feeling more laid back.

'In a way it is still about winning. But now it's not about winning his money back, now he is winning his family back, and with that will come other experiences and other changes. Perhaps we might go so far as to say he is in a sense winning his life back, though that may be too far, he already had a life, it was just that it had started to become problematic.

'And that's just it. Problematic living. Problematic lifestyles. When a person begins to experience that what they are doing is causing problems, and they can feel the effects of those problems, then they will be ready to change. Person-centred counselling offers an opportunity for people to engage with their feelings about their lifestyles and the effects of their choices. Not everyone wants that, it can be uncomfortable. Not everyone wants to change. They want to live their own lives, make their own decisions. And yet somewhere in there is the need for responsibility. Yes, people are free to make choices, but what happens when foreseeable problems occur? Some people will be unsympathetic, others will want to help them see things differently and learn from what has happened, some will want to rush in and rescue them, often leaving the old ways of thinking and feeling in existence to re-assert themselves at a later date.

'The person-centred approach is revolutionary although I prefer to think of it as "evolutionary". It says, quite clearly, that we need to offer a particular climate of relationship and trust the client's inner process of being – the actualising tendency – to urge them towards more satisfying experiences, satisfying to an increasingly fuller sense of self and congruent experiencing and expression. The urge to change may be present, along with an urge not to change. All parts need to be offered the same quality of warm acceptance and empathic sensitivity. The idea that a service for problem gamblers focuses on what the person chooses to bring rather than on what the service deems the client should talk about challenges notions of specific psychological treatments for specific conditions. It brings the fundamental human and relational factors to the fore. And rightly so.

'I have digressed a little. About Rob, I'm optimistic. He's making significant inner changes that are beginning to be reflected in outer behaviour change, and he is getting experiential feedback that is encouraging him to continue with this process. Where it will lead, I do not know. I do not need some end goal to work towards. Time will tell. All I know is that he is establishing some firm foundations for his future life and I am pleased to be playing a part in that process.'

Rob reflects on his counselling experience

Rob's reflections – 'Feels strange being asked to say something about my experience so far. And I say so far. I've really begun to get into this counselling lark. I can feel the difference in myself. It isn't easy. Not what I expected. Thought I'd be told what to do, given a list almost of things to change and how to do it. But there was nothing like that. Thank God! I mean, at the time I think that was what I wanted, but now, well, no, I've needed to change, me, how I think, how I feel. Betting, yeah, that's a problem, or it was. But there were other problems, I can see that, particularly at home. Getting myself sorted there, that's been important. I guess both that and the betting have sort of, well, I see them as being connected now. Didn't before. Separated them I suppose, and I was separating them more and more, putting the betting first. Didn't consciously think that was what I was doing, but that was what was happening.

'Funny really, one minute I'm talking about playing like a kid with Harry, then I'm sort of thinking that in a way I'm perhaps growing up. Weird that. Seems like a contradiction. Being a kid and growing up at the same time. But that's what I've had to do. It's right however daft it sounds. I couldn't talk to the guys at work about this, they'd laugh, wouldn't understand. Kenny does, he can see it. So it's good to talk to him. He's a family man, got things under control. Could do a lot worse than be like him. Sense of family, that's what he's got. That's what I'm getting.

'So, not sure what else to say. I suppose I'll carry on seeing Pat for a while. Not sure what else I'll talk about, though. Quite surprised myself talking about my childhood, stuff like that. But it felt good. Just having someone there, someone listening, really listening, not judging you, not full of airs and graces. Can't be doing with that. I like someone to be straight, say it as it is. Pat's like that, or at least that's how he feels to me. They didn't tell me what to say in this piece. Well, Pat's always steered clear of giving advice, so at least he's consistent. I guess the other thing that I want to say is that I'm very aware of Pat being there, even when I'm in my own thoughts. You'd think it would put you off, having someone sitting there looking at you. But it doesn't. Felt a bit odd to begin with, mark you. Couldn't sort of get into it. Felt easier when it was more chatty. That's something maybe counsellors should think about, be a bit more chatty. Might have helped me settle in a bit quicker. It's not like a normal conversation, and that's the way most of us have learned to talk with people. So, yeah, bit more chatty, that would have been good, particularly early on.

'You know, I still don't really know how much Pat knows about gambling and betting. I sort of think he knows a bit but he's not letting on. I'd have thought that would have mattered. But now, well, no, it doesn't. I've got to know him, respect him for what he does, how he is. It's like he's someone I could imagine sharing a couple of pints with. Some people you can't imagine that. Don't know that I'd have got on with them the same if they'd been my counsellor. I think you need someone who can speak your language. Not sure what I mean by that, maybe it's a class thing, don't know. You've got to have a counsellor you can relate to, otherwise, what's the point?

'So, yeah, I'm going to carry on working at it. Got more reasons to now. Since the last session we've learned that Karen's pregnant. Funny, I sort of feel different to how I did when she was pregnant with Harry. Don't know if it's a boy or a girl yet. But that means I'm going to have to be a bit more responsible. I'll get there. I sort of know it now. I've got reasons for change. Came too close to losing too much, maybe might have lost everything. Makes me feel a bit choked thinking that. Hadn't been thinking about that, just suddenly, there it was. Getting things in perspective, that's what I've done. Family, that's important to me now. Betting, yeah, course I enjoy it, but not like I did. It's not so important any more. It was the centre of my life. Now, well, now it's off centre, where it should be. That's it really. Not much else to say. Yeah, think I would bet on myself now to get things sorted. Don't know what odds I'd get! I think they're shortening all the time.'

Author's epilogue

Life's a gamble. We are constantly balancing risks as we make choices and decisions. Life is uncertain. We try to stack the odds in our favour. We try to make it feel more certain even though in reality it isn't. It's human nature. Where does it all begin? The child watching raindrops rolling down a window and wondering which will reach the bottom first, trying to guess? Or, maybe the question of whether someone will come when I cry? Standing up on two legs is a risky business. "I want to do it, I'm being encouraged to do it, but will I fall over." "Maybe if I hold someone's hands it will be easier, the odds will be stacked in my favour." Not that the thinking is going to be so word-dominated. There's an instinct involved. Later, maybe, the words will be there. "Can I peddle my bike without stabilisers and not fall off?" All through life we are taking risks and taking gambles. So it's not surprising that gambling and betting are such a significant feature of the human experience.

I've enjoyed writing this book. I've felt for the characters, Max and Rob as they have sought to make sense of their lives – past, present and future. Both had different life experiences and for their own reasons took to gambling and betting. Each attributed his own meaning to his gambling and betting experience and behaviour. And that's the point. People are different. People choose behaviours for particular reasons – sometimes consciously, sometimes they emerge out of an instinct, and often they are conditioned from past experiences or present expectations. Sometimes they emerge from a reaction to a specific situation, sometimes they build up over time.

The person-centred counsellor is interested in understanding what the client thinks, feels, experiences and in conveying that understanding along with a warm acceptance for the client, irrespective of what they may disclose. What purpose does gambling or betting serve in a person's life? What does it mean to them? Without it, what would they be losing? What might it mask – take it away and what is left? What motivates change, and what holds them back from change? What makes a person want to continue with a gambling or betting habit in spite of it causing problems? And what if the problems are to others, but they don't experience it as a problem?

Gambling or betting only really becomes a problem in an experiential sense for the gambler when they feel uncomfortable as a result of what they are doing and the effects it is having. It is arguably not a problem until that discomfort is present. That may be an emotional discomfort, but it could be more thoughtful. Wherever it is focused, it needs to be present for the person to begin to want to change, or, even before that, begin to just think that maybe, perhaps, something needs to be different.

Many young people are being conditioned into a more intense and widespread climate of gambling. What the result of that will be for the future is down to speculation. But I don't think it is unreasonable to conclude that the more opportunity there is for gambling, the more it will exist, and the higher the risk that people will be lured into it more deeply, and for a large number of reasons. The gambling industry wants to attract new people and it must therefore make sure that it offers what people are looking for: the promise of the big win; enough small wins to keep them tantalised and hopeful; excitement, glitz, stimulation of the senses; a sense that they are buying a product; the experience that the gambling process is separated from awareness of money being spent; opportunities to begin small and to work up, bigger stakes, bigger wins – is that any different to being lured from soft to hard drugs?

And yet people have a right to make their own choices. Yes. And people must take responsibility for those choices. They also need to be able to stand up to seductive advertising. That is not something taught in schools, it seems. We're a consumer society so we must learn to be consumers, and we have been told that the more we consume, the happier we will be. And now we are perhaps learning the somewhat painful lesson that this is a lie. Betting or gambling more doesn't make us happier. And, as we have seen from some of the disastrous changes of lifestyle amongst the very big lottery winners, winning isn't always the bed of roses it's made out to be. I don't know how many people have said to me they'd rather there were more, smaller lottery prizes, maybe one million maximum, enough to make a real difference to someone's life, but not enough so that it is simply too much to cope with.

Gambling is about ideas, the idea that we will feel different if we win, and that it will last. But it doesn't. The problem gambler needs to win again, re-live the experience, chase it down, again and again. It gives people an experience. That's what is being bought. That's the real product, an experience, a feel-good factor, or at least, the promise of it. For some people the thrill of betting or gambling is enough, winning is seen as a bonus, for others winning is the focus.

I hope this book has contributed to your having a clearer idea of the application of the person-centred approach to working with people who have gambling or betting habits that have become problematic. Both Clive and Pat, the two counsellors, made mistakes and needed to discuss their process in supervision. Counselling is a lifelong process of learning, and for the person-centred counsellor the learning is very much focused on themselves as they seek to ensure they can bring themselves congruently into relationship with their clients whilst ensuring empathic sensitivity and an ability to feel and communicate experienced warmth and acceptance of their clients. At times it feels like I am saying the same thing, again and again, juggling the words around each time. Yet we cannot avoid the essential nature of person-centred counselling and the fact that person-centred supervision is primarily concerned with ensuring that the therapist is able to offer the therapeutic conditions to their clients.

The two scenarios in this book covered many areas. There are other forms of gambling that could be addressed, of course – such as bingo. Both clients were male. Was that a stereotyping of gambling and betting? Do women gamble for different reasons or in different ways to men? How much is transferable? Will we see different betting patterns emerge amongst women with the advent of Internet gambling? And there is the growth in Internet gaming, perhaps another subtle – or not so subtle – conditioning of people into seeking particular forms of excitement. Betting on the outcomes for these games may already be happening, and if it isn't then I'm sure it won't be long before it is introduced.

I have a genuine concern that people are being conditioned into an expanding betting and gambling culture. I don't want it banned. As I've said, it is an instinctive aspect to the human experience. There will always be gambling and betting, it can be fun, it does give us a range of experiences and these can feel very satisfying. But it can be exploited and people can be damaged. If these effects can be minimised then surely in civilised society this should be the major goal.

I am convinced that the coming years and decades will see counsellors working with more and more clients with gambling problems. I cannot imagine it being otherwise, and with gambling habits ingrained from earlier ages. I want to see the person-centred approach being recognised as a credible response both as a form of therapy, and as a wider set of values and principles that a society needs to adopt, or at least be mindful of.

Person-centred theory affirms the importance of congruence, of being genuine, authentic, transparent, and at a time when the world seems to be embracing quite the opposite. It seems to me that the relational component of the person-centred approach, based on the presence of the core conditions, is emerging strongly as a counter to the sense of isolation that frequently accompanies deep psychological and emotional problems, and which is a feature of materialistic societies. It is fascinating that this is occurring now given that the concept of relational counselling was very much a driving force in the early development of the ideas that then developed into what we know as the person-centred approach. Of the counselling relationship Rogers wrote in 1942:

> The counselling relationship is one in which warmth of acceptance and absence of any coercion or personal pressure on the part of the counsellor permits the maximum expression of feelings, attitudes, and problems by the counselee . . . In the unique experience of complete emotional freedom within a well-defined framework the client is free to recognize and understand his impulses and patterns, positive and negative, as in no other relationship (Rogers, 1942, pp. 113–14).

Working with a person or client who has a gambling problem, like working with any other client about any other issue, is about forming therapeutic relationship and offering the client time and a space in which to explore, with increasing openness and authenticity, what they are experiencing. The person-centred counsellor will not take the perspective of being there to 'treat problem gambling', but to form a therapeutic relationship that will enable that client to experience constructive personality change that is self-directed through the process of the actualising tendency. As they become more authentically aware of themselves, and diminish the effects of 'conditions of worth' and re-evaluate their sense of self, they will very likely seek to change behaviours so as to establish new ones that more closely satisfy the needs of their changing sense of self. As the causes of their problematic gambling are recognised and understood, and begin to loosen their grip, the gambling behaviour will change, and with a likelihood that it will be in a sustainable way because it is driven by psychological and emotional change which, itself, is the result of the actualising tendency operating within a person-centred therapeutic experience.

Appendix

'Cycle of change' model

Another way of approaching change is to take a more cognitive-behavioural perspective and to focus specifically on the behaviour that is being changed and the attitude of the person towards that behaviour. The 'cycle of change' model, devised in the early 1980s by two American psychologists Prochaska and DiClemente (1982), describes the process and stages people pass through when undergoing change in terms of behaviour and attitude towards that behaviour, and ways of working to encourage them to change. It was originally devised in relation to smoking, but has been widely applied to working with people who have addictive behaviours – for instance, in relation to drug and alcohol use. Recently, one of its co-authors has produced his own book (DiClemente, 2003), which offers a more detailed description of the application of this model in treating addiction. The 'cycle of change' model suggests that people pass through stages and each stage has certain characteristics and demands particular areas of focus and response in order to help the client move on. The stages are as follow:

- pre-contemplation
- contemplation
- preparation
- action
- maintenance
- lapse or relapse.

Pre-contemplation

In the stage of *pre-contemplation*, the client will not be thinking about change. This may because they simply do not see their gambling as a problem or as something needing to be addressed. It could be that they do recognise that it has become an issue, but find the idea of change too difficult or uncomfortable to consider and have pushed the idea aside, choosing to ignore it and carry on as they have been. This might be described as denial, although it is worth acknowledging that this stage is not as negative as is sometimes made out. Being in denial when someone is aware that there is a problem, and which they are uncomfortable about but seeking to push the discomfort aside, means that the client is in a state of incongruence. Incongruence, as we have seen, is one of the necessary conditions for constructive personality change. If the person-centred counsellor can offer warm and genuine acceptance of the client's need to deny the difficulty, and can empathise with that behaviour and the resulting discomfort, change may happen. Often the pushing away of a problem is a psychological reflex, and when it is explored within a supportive therapeutic climate, it can be broken down and/or re-evaluated, with the possibility of a different outcome.

Contemplation

At the *contemplation* stage, the client is, in a sense, more in touch with, and accepting of, their discomfort about, in this context, their gambling, and is entering into a process of thinking about change, exploring it and weighing it up. This can be a lengthy process. People can, and do, take time to make decisions that involve change, particularly changes that affect them directly and intimately as a person. Social behaviours are important to people, along with a sense of winning. It will not necessarily be changed easily and quickly, and may involve a good deal of exploration and heart-searching. The process cannot be hurried. The client needs time to genuinely weigh up the pros and cons of change, and to really understand, for themselves, what they might be embarking upon and why.

It is the stage at which a client may be keeping a diary of their gambling to understand the quantity, pattern and type of gambling undertaken, to help get an objective picture. Also, the triggers for gambling may be identified. It is a time for the person to really get as full an understanding of their gambling pattern and the meanings that they attach to it as possible. The latter is important and can get overlooked where there is a rush made towards behaviour change. The gambling experience can mean many things to different people, and particular forms of gambling may have particular meanings, for instance, a lone gambler on the Internet may not be seeking the same social experience as the person sitting playing black jack in the casino, meeting friends and experiencing a sense of status and value in himself from the experience. The person betting at the races may be part of a social group, or they may be very much an individual for whom the same social element is less important. A particular gambler may have a range of gambling activities, each being chosen for different reasons, perhaps in response to specific configurations, or sub-configurations of the dominating gambling configuration within that individual's structure of self. All of this is important to recognise so that the client can be as fully informed as possible as they weigh up the options and seek to understand themselves and what drives the urge to engage in particular gambling behaviours. This information embraces both the client as a person and the gambling patterns.

During contemplation a client may decide, for whatever reason, not to pursue change. They will have reasons for this, and these must also be warmly and genuinely accepted. Sometimes, as a result of this acceptance, the client may revisit the process and change their mind, others will not. They may break from the counselling, or may wish to stay in the counselling relationship perhaps to work on another issue. At least if the client chooses not to change, it is possible that their perspective on the problem will have changed and, given different circumstances at a future point, they may draw on this to make changes.

Preparation

The contemplation stage is also helping the client to inform themselves in readiness for the phase of *preparation*. At this point the client will have recognised that, yes, on balance, they want to make changes and they will begin to plan their strategy. They will formulate their goals – and it is important that they are owned by the client, and are realistic. Too many people lapse because goals are unrealistic, having been set more from the agenda of the counsellor than the client. The client has got to feel that whatever goal they set themselves is realistic and attainable. They also need to have a clear time-frame to work within, again which must be owned and be realistic to the client. In terms of a gambling pattern, this could involve reducing or cutting out particular types of gambling, reducing the amount staked and the frequency of the gambling behaviour.

Some clients will aim for abstinence, others for a more 'controlled gambling' regime. Also, there will perhaps be an element of 'harm minimisation': a useful term which means to reduce the harm – for instance economic, marital – that stems from the gambling habit.

Risks of a lapse or relapse are also discussed, and ways of minimising them, or of responding to them, are planned. It is better to have ideas formulated in order to avoid a slip in the abstinence or controlled gambling regime, rather than have to try and find a solution afterwards. A person will feel good about achieving an avoidance of a lapse, and this can be built on to enhance motivation.

Action

Having created the strategy for change it then has to be put into *action*. Quite simply, this is the stage at which the plan is enacted. Support systems will now be in place as well as systems to enable the client to self-monitor. The client may continue to keep a diary of their gambling pattern, what was gambled, how, where, with whom, what was the effect – winnings/losses, and emotions. However, whilst reducing the amount of money lost through gambling may be an eventual aim, this can become a barrier to achieving a change in the gambling pattern. Yes, it can be a motivating factor, but if the amount lost is not reduced, it can sap the client's motivation. For some clients, simply focusing on a more healthy lifestyle – introducing other areas of interest and social experience, or a reduction in quantity without too much emphasis on the financial aspect – can be helpful. Sometimes, the early stages of change simply require the breaking up of the pattern that is established, helping the person to begin to appreciate that they have choices, that they can decide to do something else, or bet less. Gambling patterns can become habitual – we gamble today what we gambled yesterday, because we gambled that way the day before. Encouraging a sense of adventure can be helpful, for changing a gambling pattern is an opportunity to experience something new. It is not always solely about giving something up. Gambling not only swallows money, it also swallows time, and there will be a real need to consider how the time can be redirected to other satisfying experiences.

Maintenance

Change must be maintained, but for how long before it is deemed a sustainable change? It will vary from person to person, and depends largely on their psychological responses to opportunities or triggers to return to their original gambling pattern. Monitoring should continue, high-risk situations should be thought through. It may take some time before the person feels that they are no longer having to make themselves avoid gambling or maintain control. The person has to pass through a psychological process of accepting themselves as a person who doesn't gamble, or gambles in a particular way, or to a certain level.

Lapse or relapse

There may be slips or blips, when more than is planned is gambled, or perhaps a particular type of gambling creeps back into the gambling pattern. These can be usefully explored. There will be a reason why, and it is likely to be associated with a feeling, an experience. It may be something identified during contemplation/preparation, but for which planning has not proved adequate. Or it may be something unexpected, requiring a process of exploration leading to informed planning as to how to deal with it should it arise again. There may be an underlying emotional issue to work through.

The task, at this stage, is to ensure that a lapse does not become a relapse. This will have been discussed in the preparation phase. Also, to ensure that the client does not break contact so that they can be encouraged to continue with their effort, if they wish to, learning from what has occurred. It can be depressing to lapse, and tempting to give up. Change is not easy, and counsellors must appreciate this.

As we have seen, there are exit points from the cycle. Clients may exit the process either in contemplation or preparation if they feel that the time is not right for change, or simply find themselves unable to sustain their motivation. They may exit the cycle from maintenance having achieved their goal, whether that is a change in the nature of the gambling habit, or the amount gambled. Finally, they may exit from lapse or relapse, going back into their previous pattern of gambling as a result of which they may choose not to try to change, or they may return to pre-contemplation to weigh up and learn from their process so far.

What is key is to bear in mind that whilst there is change taking place in gambling behaviour, this has to be underpinned by a psychological process of change. The person-centred counsellor does not direct the client around the model, it exists to inform the process. Clients often find it interesting to have a handout so they can think, for themselves, what the different stages mean to them. They may see different stages, or want to use their own language to define their process. All of this is perfectly reasonable and acceptable. But the psychological process of change must not be lost sight of in the rush to achieve behaviour modification. Gradual and informed change, sustained over time, at the client's pace and to the client's agenda, is more valuable than a cycle of constant failure which can be psychologically debilitating, and undermining of the person.

References

Bozarth J (1998) *Person-Centred Therapy: a revolutionary paradigm*. PCCS Books, Ross-on-Wye.

Bozarth J and Wilkins P (eds) (2001) *Rogers' Therapeutic Conditions: evolution, theory and practice*. Volume 3: *Congruence*. PCCS Books, Ross-on-Wye.

Bryant-Jefferies R (2003) *Time Limited Therapy in Primary Care: a person-centred dialogue*. Radcliffe Medical Press, Oxford.

Bryant-Jefferies R (2005) *Person-centred Counselling Supervision: personal and professional*. Radcliffe Publishing, Oxford.

DiClemente CC (2003) *Addiction and Change*. The Guilford Press, New York.

DiClemente CC and Prochaska JO (1998) Towards a comprehensive, transtheoretical model of change: stages of change and addictive behaviours. In: W Miller and N Heather (eds) *Treating Addictive Behaviours* (2e). Plenum, New York.

Embleton Tudor L, Keemar K, Tudor K *et al*. (2004) *The Person-Centred Approach: a contemporary introduction*. Palgrave MacMillan, Basingstoke.

Evans R (1975) *Carl Rogers: the man and his ideas*. Dutton and Co., New York.

Fisher SE (1992) Measuring pathological gambling in children. The case of fruit machines in the UK. *Journal of Gambling Studies*. **8**: 263–85.

Fisher SE (1993) The pull of the fruit machine: a sociological typology of young players. *Sociological Review*. **41**: 446–74.

Fisher SE and Bellringer P (1997) *The Young Fruit Machine Player*. Forum on Young People and Gambling, London.

Gaylin N (2001) *Family, Self and Psychotherapy: a person-centred perspective*. PCCS Books, Ross-on-Wye.

Griffiths MD (1991a) Amusement machine playing in childhood and adolescence: a comparative analysis of video games and fruit machines. *Journal of Adolescence*. **14**: 53–73.

Griffiths MD (1991b) The observational analysis of adolescent gambling in UK amusement arcades. *Journal of Community and Applied Social Psychology*. **1**: 309–20.

Griffiths MD (1995) *Adolescent Gambling*. Routledge, London.

Griffiths MD (2002) *Gambling and Gaming Addictions in Adolescence*. BPS Blackwell, Oxford.

Griffiths MD and Sutherland I (1998) Adolescent gambling and drug use. *Journal of Community and Applied Social Psychology*. **8**: 423–7.

Haugh S and Merry T (eds) (2001) *Rogers' Therapeutic Conditions: evolution, theory and practice*. Volume 2: *Empathy*. PCCS Books, Ross-on-Wye.

Home Office (2001) *Gaming Review Report*. HMSO, London.

Kirschenbaum H (2005) The current status of Carl Rogers and the person-centred approach. *Psychotherapy*. **42**(1): 37–51.

Mearns D and Thorne B (1988) *Person-Centred Counselling in Action*. Sage, London.

Mearns D and Thorne B (1999) *Person-Centred Counselling in Action* (2e). Sage, London.

Mearns D and Thorne B (2000) *Person-Centred Therapy Today*. Sage, London.

Merry T (2001) Congruence and the supervision of client-centred therapists. In: G Wyatt (ed.) *Rogers' Therapeutic Conditions: evolution, theory and practice*. Volume 1: *Congruence*. PCCS Books, Ross-on-Wye, pp. 174–83.

Merry T (2002) *Learning and Being in Person-Centred Counselling* (2e). PCCS Books, Ross-on-Wye.

Moore SM and Ohtsuka K (1997) Gambling activities of young Australians: developing a model of behaviour. *Journal of Gambling Studies*. **13**(3): 207–36.

Patterson CH (2000) *Understanding Psychotherapy: fifty years of client-centred theory and practice*. PCCS Books, Ross-on-Wye.

Prochaska JO and DiClemente CC (1982) Transtheoretical therapy: towards a more integrative model of change. *Psychotherapy: theory, research and practice*. **19**: 276–88.

Rogers CR (1942) *Counselling and Psychotherapy: newer concepts in practice*. Houghton-Mifflin Co., Boston, MA.

Rogers CR (1951) *Client-Centred Therapy*. Constable, London.

Rogers CR (1957) The necessary and sufficient conditions of therapeutic personality change. *Journal of Consulting Psychology*. **21**: 95–103.

Rogers CR (1959) A theory of therapy, personality and interpersonal relationships as developed in the client-centred framework. In: S Koch (ed.) *Psychology: a study of a science*. Volume 3: *Formulations of the Person and the Social Context*. McGraw-Hill, New York, pp. 185–246.

Rogers CR (1967) *On Becoming a Person*. Constable, London. (Original work published in 1961.)

Rogers CR (1980) *A Way of Being*. Houghton-Mifflin Co., Boston, MA.

Rogers CR (1986) A client-centered/person-centered approach to therapy. In: I Kutash and A Wolfe (eds) *Psychotherapists' Casebook*. Jossey Bass, San Francisco, CA, pp. 236–57.

Sproston KB, Erens B and Orford J (2000) *Gambling Behaviour in Britain: results from the British Gambling Prevalence Survey*. National Centre for Social Research, London.

Tudor K and Worrall M (2004) *Freedom to Practise: person-centred approaches to supervision*. PCCS Books, Ross-on-Wye.

Warner M (2002) Psychological contact, meaningful process and human nature. In: G Wyatt and P Sanders (eds) *Rogers' Therapeutic Conditions: evolution, theory and practice*. Volume 4: *Contact and Perception*. PCCS Books, Ross-on-Wye, pp. 76–95.

Wilkins P (2003) *Person-Centred Therapy in Focus*. Sage, London.

Winters KC, Stinchfield R, Fulkerson J (1993) Patterns and characteristics of adolescent gambling. *Journal of Gambling Studies*. 9(4): 371–87.

Wood RTA and Griffiths MD (1998) The acquisition, development and maintenance of lottery and scratchcard gambling in adolescence. *Journal of Adolescence*. 21: 265–73.

Wyatt G (ed.) (2001) *Rogers' Therapeutic Conditions: evolution, theory and practice*. Volume 1: *Congruence*. PCCS Books, Ross-on-Wye.

Wyatt G and Sanders P (eds) (2002) *Rogers' Therapeutic Conditions: evolution, theory and practice*. Volume 4: *Contact and Perception*. PCCS Books, Ross-on-Wye.

Useful contacts

Person-centred

Association for the Development of the Person-Centered Approach (ADPCA)
Email: adpca-web@signs.portents.com
Website: www.adpca.org

An international association, with members in 27 countries, for those interested in the development of client-centred therapy and the person-centred approach.

British Association for the Person-Centred Approach (BAPCA)
Bm-BAPCA
London WC1N 3XX
Tel: 01989 770948
Email: info@bapca.org.uk
Website: www.bapca.org.uk

National association promoting the person-centred approach. Publishes a regular newsletter *Person-to-Person* and promotes awareness of person-centred events and issues in the UK.

Person-Centred Therapy Scotland
Tel: 0870 7650871
Email: info@pctscotland.co.uk
Website: www.pctscotland.co.uk

An association of person-centred therapists in Scotland which offers training and networking opportunities to members, with the aim of fostering high standards of professional practice.

World Association for Person-Centred and Experiential Psychotherapy and Counselling
Email: secretariat@pce-world.org
Website: www.pce-world.org

The association aims to provide a worldwide forum for those professionals in science and practice who are committed to, and embody in their work, the theoretical principles of the person-centred approach first postulated by Carl Rogers. The association publishes *Person-centred and Experiential Psychotherapies*, an international journal which 'creates a dialogue among different parts of the person-centred/experiential therapy tradition, supporting, informing and challenging academics and practitioners with the aim of the development of these approaches in a broad professional, scientific and political context'.

Problem gambling

Gam-Anon
National Service Office
PO Box 88
London SW10 0EU
Helpline: 08700 50 88 80
Email: contact@gamanon.org.uk
Website: www.gamanon.org.uk

Gamblers Anonymous
PO Box 88
London SW10 0EU
Helpline: 08700 50 88 80
Website: www.gamblersanonymous.org.uk

GamCare
GamCare
2&3 Baden Place
Crosby Row
London SE1 1YW
Tel: 020 7378 5200
Fax: 020 7378 5237
Helpline: 0845 6000 133 (24 hour, 7 days a week)
Email: info@gamcare.org.uk
Website: www.gamcare.org.uk

GamCare is a registered charity and has become the leading authority on the provision of information, advice and practical help in addressing the social impact of gambling. It strives to develop strategies that will:

- improve the understanding of the social impact of gambling
- promote a responsible approach to gambling
- address the needs of those adversely affected by a gambling dependency.

GamCare takes a non-judgemental approach on gambling. It does not wish to restrict the choices or opportunities for anyone to operate or engage in gambling opportunities that are available legally and operated responsibly.

The National Council on Problem Gambling
216 G Street NE, Suite 200
Washington, DC 20002
Tel: 1–202–547–9204
Fax: 1–202–547–9206
Email: ncpg@ncpgambling.org
Website: www.ncpgambling.org

Index